T0362396

Perioperative Management of the Thoracic Surgery Patient

Editors

VIRGINIA R. LITLE
ROBERT J. CANELLI

THORACIC
SURGERY CLINICS

www.thoracic.theclinics.com

Consulting Editor
VIRGINIA R. LITLE

August 2020 • Volume 30 • Number 3

ELSEVIER

1600 John F. Kennedy Boulevard • Suite 1800 • Philadelphia, Pennsylvania, 19103-2899

http://www.thoracic.theclinics.com

THORACIC SURGERY CLINICS Volume 30, Number 3
August 2020 ISSN 1547-4127, ISBN-13: 978-0-323-73301-4

Editor: John Vassallo (j.vassallo@elsevier.com)
Developmental Editor: Laura Fisher

Thoracic Surgery Clinics (ISSN 1547-4127) is published quarterly by Elsevier Inc., 360 Park Avenue South, New York, NY 10010-1710. Months of publication are February, May, August, and November. Business and editorial offices: 1600 John F. Kennedy Boulevard, Suite 1800, Philadelphia, PA 19103-2899. Periodicals postage paid at New York, NY, and additional mailing offices. Subscription prices are $393.00 per year (US individuals), $623.00 per year (US institutions), $100.00 per year (US students), $460.00 per year (Canadian individuals), $806.00 per year (Canadian institutions), $100.00 per year (Canadian students), $225.00 per year (international students), $480.00 per year (international individuals), and $806.00 per year (international institu-tions). Foreign air speed delivery is included in all Clinics' subscription prices. All prices are subject to change without notice. **POSTMASTER:** Send address changes to Thoracic Surgery Clinics, Elsevier Health Sciences Division, Subscription Customer Service, 3251 Riverport Lane, Maryland Heights, MO 63043. **Customer Service (orders, claims, online, change of address): Telephone: 1-800-654-2452 (U.S. and Canada); 314-447-8871 (outside U.S. and Canada). Fax: 314-447-8029. E-mail: jour-nalscustomerservice-usa@elsevier.com (for print support); journalsonlinesupport-usa@elsevier.com (for online support).**

Reprints. For copies of 100 or more, of articles in this publication, please contact Commercial Rights Department, Elsevier Inc., 360 Park Avenue South, New York, NY 10010-1710. Tel: 212-633-3874; Fax: 212-633-3820; E-mail: reprints@elsevier.com.

Thoracic Surgery Clinics is covered in *MEDLINE/PubMed (Index Medicus), EMBASE/Excerpta Medica, Science Citation Index Expanded (SciSearch®), Journal Citation Reports/Science Edition,* and *Current Contents®/Clinical Medicine.*

Contributors

CONSULTING EDITOR

VIRGINIA R. LITLE, MD
Professor, Department of Surgery, Chief,
Division of Thoracic Surgery, Boston
University,Boston, Massachusetts, USA

EDITORS

VIRGINIA R. LITLE, MD
Professor, Department of Surgery, Chief,
Division of Thoracic Surgery, Boston
University,Boston, Massachusetts, USA

ROBERT J. CANELLI, MD
Assistant Professor of Anesthesiology, Boston
University School of Medicine,
Anesthesiologist and Intensivist, Boston
Medical Center, Boston, Massachusetts, USA

AUTHORS

RANDAL S. BLANK, MD, PhD
Professor, Division of General Anesthesiology,
Department of Anesthesiology, University of
Virginia Health System, Charlottesville,
Virginia, USA

LISA M. BROWN, MD, MAS
Section of General Thoracic Surgery,
Department of Surgery, University of California,
Davis Health, Sacramento, California, USA

MATTHEW BYLER, MD, MBA
Surgical Resident, Division of Thoracic and
Cardiovascular Surgery, Department of
Surgery, University of Virginia Health System,
Charlottesville, Virginia, USA

ROBERT CANELLI, MD
Assistant Professor of Anesthesiology, Boston
University School of Medicine,
Anesthesiologist and Intensivist, Boston
Medical Center, Boston, Massachusetts,
USA

ROBERT J. CERFOLIO, MD, MBA
Executive Vice President, Vice Dean, Chief of
Hospital Operations, Professor of
Cardiothoracic Surgery, Department of

Cardiothoracic Surgery, NYU Langone Health,
New York, New York, USA

JAMES M. CLARK, MD
Section of General Thoracic Surgery,
Department of Surgery, University of
California, Davis Health, Sacramento,
California, USA

DAVID T. COOKE, MD
Section of General Thoracic Surgery,
Department of Surgery, University of
California, Davis Health, Sacramento,
California, USA

LISA COOPER, MD
Division of Aging, Brigham and Women's
Hospital, Boston, Massachusetts, USA

AARON R. DEZUBE, MD
Division of Thoracic Surgery, Brigham and
Women's Hospital, Boston, Massachusetts,
USA

TRAVIS C. GERACI, MD
Fellow, Department of Cardiothoracic Surgery,
NYU Langone Health, New York, New York,
USA

ANDRE F. GOSLING, MD
Department of Anesthesia, Critical Care and Pain Medicine, Beth Israel Deaconess Medical Center, Boston, Massachusetts, USA

NATHAN HAYWOOD, MD
Surgical Resident, Division of Thoracic and Cardiovascular Surgery, Department of Surgery, University of Virginia Health System, Charlottesville, Virginia, USA

MICHAEL T. JAKLITSCH, MD
Division of Thoracic Surgery, Brigham and Women's Hospital, Boston, Massachusetts, USA

WALKER JULLIARD, MD
Thoracic Surgery Fellow, Division of Thoracic and Cardiovascular Surgery, Department of Surgery, University of Virginia Health System, Charlottesville, Virginia, USA

HARDEEP S. KALSI, MBBs, IBSc
Division of Medicine, Lungs for Living Research Centre, UCL Respiratory, University College London, London, United Kingdom

MICHAEL S. KENT, MD
Division of Thoracic Surgery and Interventional Pulmonology, Beth Israel Deaconess Medical Center, Boston, Massachusetts, USA

VIRGINIA R. LITLE, MD
Professor, Department of Surgery, Chief, Division of Thoracic Surgery, Boston University, Boston, Massachusetts, USA

JAMES D. LUKETICH, MD, FACS
Henry T. Bahnson Professor of Cardiothoracic Surgery, Chairman, Department of Cardiothoracic Surgery, Chief, Division of Thoracic and Foregut Surgery, Department of Cardiothoracic Surgery Director, Thoracic Surgical Oncology, Director, UPMC Esophageal and Lung Surgery Institute, Director, Mark Ravitch/Leon C. Hirsch Center for Minimally Invasive Surgery, University of Pittsburgh Medical Center, University of Pittsburgh School of Medicine, Pittsburgh, Pennsylvania, USA

BRENT LURIA, MD
Clinical Associate Professor, Department of Anesthesiology, NYU Langone Health, New York, New York, USA

KYLE MARSHALL, MD
Assistant Professor of Anesthesiology, University of Colorado Anschutz Medical Campus, Aurora, Colorado, USA

LINDA W. MARTIN, MD, MPH
Associate Professor, Division of Thoracic and Cardiovascular Surgery, Department of Surgery, University of Virginia Health System, Charlottesville, Virginia, USA

THEOFILOS MATHEOS, MD
Assistant Professor of Anesthesiology and Surgery, Division of Critical Care Medicine, Medical Director of Pre-Surgical Evaluation Clinic, Department of Anesthesiology and Perioperative Medicine, University of Massachusetts Medical School, UMass Memorial Medical Center, Worcester, Massachusetts, USA

KELEIGH McLAUGHLIN, MD
CA-3 Resident in Anesthesiology, University of Colorado Anschutz Medical Campus, Aurora, Colorado, USA

THOMAS J. MELVIN, MD
Department of Surgery, University of Pittsburgh Medical Center Mercy Hospital, Pittsburgh, Pennsylvania, USA

NEAL NAVANI, MD, MSc, PhD
Division of Medicine, Lungs for Living Research Centre, UCL Respiratory, University College London, London, United Kingdom

IAN NICKEL, MD
Surgical Resident, Division of Thoracic and Cardiovascular Surgery, Department of Surgery, University of Virginia Health System, Charlottesville, Virginia, USA

MORIHITO OKADA, MD, PhD
Professor of Surgery, Department of Surgical Oncology, Hiroshima University, Hiroshima City, Hiroshima, Japan

LAKSHMI RAM, MD
Surgical Critical Care Fellow, Department of Anesthesiology, Division of Critical Care, UMass Memorial Medical Center, Worcester, Massachusetts, USA

GERARDO RODRIGUEZ, MD
Associate Medical Director, Surgical Intensive Care Unit, Clinical Associate Professor of Anesthesiology and Surgery, Boston University School of Medicine, Boston Medical Center, Boston, Massachusetts, USA

INDERPAL S. SARKARIA, MD, MBA, FACS
Assistant Professor of Cardiothoracic Surgery, Vice Chair, Clinical Affairs, Director of Thoracic Robotic Surgery, Co-Director, UPMC Esophageal Surgery Institute, Department of Cardiothoracic Surgery, University of Pittsburgh Medical Center, University of Pittsburgh School of Medicine, Pittsburgh, Pennsylvania, USA

PRABHU SASANKAN, BS
NYU Grossman School of Medicine, NYU Langone Health, New York, New York, USA

ERIK SCOTT, MD
Surgical Resident, Division of Thoracic and Cardiovascular Surgery, Department of Surgery, University of Virginia Health System, Charlottesville, Virginia, USA

SHAHZAD SHAEFI, MD, MPH
Department of Anesthesia, Critical Care and Pain Medicine, Beth Israel Deaconess Medical Center, Boston, Massachusetts, USA

MELINA SHONI, MD
Resident Physician, Department of Anesthesiology, Boston Medical Center, Boston, Massachusetts, USA

PRAVEEN SRIDHAR, MD
General Surgery Resident, Division of Thoracic Surgery, Department of Surgery, Boston Medical Center, Boston University School of Medicine, Surgical Education Office, Boston, Massachusetts, USA

KEI SUZUKI, MD
Assistant Professor of Surgery, Division of Thoracic Surgery, Department of Surgery, Boston Medical Center, Boston University School of Medicine, Boston, Massachusetts, USA

RICKY THAKRAR, MBBs, PhD, IBSc
Division of Medicine, Lungs for Living Research Centre, UCL Respiratory, University College London, London, United Kingdom

AMMARA A. WATKINS, MD, MPH
Division of Thoracic Surgery and Interventional Pulmonology, Beth Israel Deaconess Medical Center, Boston, Massachusetts, USA

JENNIFER L. WILSON, MD, MPH
Division of Thoracic Surgery and Interventional Pulmonology, Beth Israel Deaconess Medical Center, Boston, Massachusetts, USA

TADEUSZ D. WITEK, MD
Department of Cardiothoracic Surgery, University of Pittsburgh Medical Center, University of Pittsburgh School of Medicine, Pittsburgh, Pennsylvania, USA

JONATHAN C. YEUNG, MD, PhD, FRCSC
Assistant Professor, Department of Surgery, University of Toronto, Toronto General Hospital, Toronto, Ontario, Canada

AIMEE ZHANG, MD
Surgical Resident, Division of Thoracic and Cardiovascular Surgery, Department of Surgery, University of Virginia Health System, Charlottesville, Virginia, USA

Contents

and open versus minimally invasive. Each approach has its associated risks and advantages. When determining the optimal approach and technique, several variables need to be considered. The key variables include patient and tumor characteristics, as well as surgeon comfort and experience with each approach. Regardless of the approach, the goal should remain the same, that is, performing a safe operation without compromise of oncologic principles.

Section II: Intraoperative Management

Interventional pulmonology is a dynamic and evolving field in respiratory medicine. Advances have improved the ability to diagnose and manage diseases of the airways. A shift toward early detection of malignant disease has generated a focus on innovative diagnostic techniques. With patient populations living longer with malignant and benign diseases, the role for interventional bronchoscopy has grown. In cancer groups, novel immunotherapies have improved the prospects of clinical outcomes and reignited a focus on optimizing patient performance status to enable access to anticancer therapy. This review discusses current and emerging diagnostic modalities and therapeutic approaches available to manage airway diseases.

Section III: Postoperative Management

Thoracic surgery is considered one of the most painful surgical procedures performed. Pain is mediated via several mechanisms and is affected by the surgical approach as well as patient factors. Pain after thoracic surgery can be debilitating and lead to poor outcomes, such as respiratory complications, longer hospital stays, poor quality of life, and chronic post-thoracotomy pain syndrome. A multimodal approach to postoperative pain that combines systemic and regional anesthesia has been shown to be the most effective in optimizing analgesia in these patients.

Prolonged air leak or alveolar-pleural fistula is common after lung resection and can usually be managed with continued pleural drainage until resolution. Further management options include blood patch administration, chemical pleurodesis, and 1-way endobronchial valve placement. Bronchopleural fistula is rare but is associated with high mortality, often caused by development of concomitant empyema. Bronchopleural fistula should be confirmed with bronchoscopy, which may allow bronchoscopic intervention; however, transthoracic stump revision or window thoracostomy may be required.

Esophagectomy is a complex operation with many potential complications. Early recognition of postoperative complications allows for the best chance for patient survival. Diagnosis and management of conduit complications, including leak, necrosis, and conduit-airway fistulae, are reviewed. Other common complications, such as chylothorax and recurrent laryngeal nerve injury, also are discussed.

THORACIC SURGERY CLINICS

SERIES OF RELATED INTEREST

Surgical Clinics
http://www.surgical.theclinics.com

Surgical Oncology Clinics
http://www.surgonc.theclinics.com

Advances in Surgery
http://www.advancessurgery.com

THE CLINICS ARE AVAILABLE ONLINE!
Access your subscription at:
www.theclinics.com

Foreword

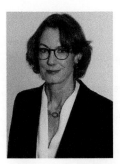

Virginia R. Litle, MD
Consulting Editor

For the past 10 years, M. Blair Marshall, MD, Consulting Editor for *Thoracic Surgery Clinics*, brought us an array of topics from surgical to professional. We are thankful to Dr Marshall for keeping us current on not only the management of benign and malignant thoracic diseases but also the technical advances for which she is an expert. I am excited to introduce myself as her successor as Consulting Editor. I look forward to working with general thoracic colleagues as well as involving specialists from other scientific and medical fields to continue the tradition of updating us all on what is topical and of interest to our thoracic audience from trainees to senior surgeons. I welcome suggestions from you all about what advances in the field you would like to learn. Our mutual goals should be to move our field forward for the sake of our patients!

Sincerely,

Virginia R. Litle, MD
Division of Thoracic Surgery
Department of Surgery
Boston University
88 East Newton Street
Collamore Building, Suite 7380
Boston, MA 02118, USA

E-mail address:
Virginia.litle@bmc.org

Twitter: @vlitlemd (V.R. Litle)

Thorac Surg Clin 30 (2020) xi
https://doi.org/10.1016/j.thorsurg.2020.06.001
1547-4127/20/© 2020 Published by Elsevier Inc.

Preface
Perioperative Management of the Thoracic Patient Continues to Evolve

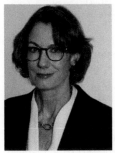
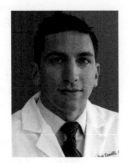

Virginia R. Litle, MD   Robert J. Canelli, MD
Editors

We are excited to bring you this focused issue for the *Thoracic Surgery Clinics* on "Perioperative Management of the Thoracic Patient." In contrast to other surgical specialties, general thoracic surgery in particular requires deliberate coordination between all members of the operative team. To optimize patient safety and operative efficiency, anesthesiologists and surgeons must communicate not only intraoperatively but also preoperatively as well. General thoracic surgeons and anesthesiologists need to know how to take an evidence-based approach to manage perioperative problems. Lung resections and esophagectomies are fraught with the overriding risks of intraoperative and postoperative complications. Mitigating risk starts with a shared decision-making conversation between patient and surgeon, once the patient elects to pursue operative therapy for their thoracic malignancy, thymic lesion, or benign esophageal disease. From the preoperative gateway, down the intraoperative path, and through discharge, the patient will travel safely with guidance from the expert contributions presented in the following pages.

Matheos and colleagues lead us off with an update on the preoperative evaluation and include an algorithm for cardiopulmonary testing. The preoperative management of thoracic patients has evolved beyond simply pulmonary function tests and the as-needed stress echocardiogram. Dezube and colleagues outline a prehabilitation program that calculates a patient's frailty index and considers physiologic versus chronologic age. Prehabilitation will optimize patients before surgery, so that they may sprint down the operative road without stumbling. Unlike Prehabilitation, which remains fairly nascent in our field, enhanced recovery after surgery (ERAS) programs have become increasingly routine in our field, perhaps because they are less resource intensive. Haywood and coauthors take us through the more immediate preoperative nutritional guidelines to the intraoperative anesthetic suggestions with the ultimate goal of reducing the patient's postoperative pain and return to homeostasis.

Intraoperative management is a component of ERAS; however, Shoni and Rodriguez discuss patient-specific ventilator management strategies and one-lung ventilation complications. For the

Thorac Surg Clin 30 (2020) xiii–xiv
https://doi.org/10.1016/j.thorsurg.2020.04.012
1547-4127/20/© 2020 Published by Elsevier Inc.

surgeons, the Pittsburgh team of Witek and colleagues offers decision trees for operative approaches, including minimally invasive versus open and choice of type of esophagectomy depending on details of patient disease. Geraci, with senior author Cerfolio, applies their extensive robotic experience to cover both surgical and anesthetic concerns for mediastinal, pulmonary, and esophageal operations. Intraoperative guidance on how to reduce postoperative complications like air leaks and anastomotic leaks is well summarized by surgical colleagues in their contributions; however, when such complications arise, Clark and colleagues and Yeung offer management options.

We have asked our contributors to delineate the steps for optimal perioperative management of the complex thoracic patient. The mutual goal of the anesthesiologists and surgeons managing patients with lung or esophagus cancer in particular is patient safety. Thank you to our contributors. We hope you will enjoy this issue!

Virginia R. Litle, MD
Division of Thoracic Surgery
Department of Surgery
88 East Newton Street
Collamore Building, Suite 7380
Boston, MA 02118, USA

Robert J. Canelli, MD
Boston Medical Center
Department of Anesthesiology
750 Albany Street, Suite 2R
Boston, MA 02118, USA

E-mail addresses:
Virginia.litle@bmc.org (V.R. Litle)
Robert.canelli@bmc.org (R.J. Canelli)

Section A: Preoperative

Preoperative Evaluation for Thoracic Surgery

Theofilos Matheos, MD[a],*, Lakshmi Ram, MD[b], Robert Canelli, MD[c]

KEYWORDS

• Thoracic preoperative evaluation • Cardiac risk stratification • Pulmonary function testing

KEY POINTS

- Readers will understand the physiologic effects of chest surgery and how intraoperative positioning can affect patient selection.
- This article discusses comorbid conditions that impact postoperative outcomes.
- Readers will review an algorithm based on pulmonary function testing that can identify surgical candidates.

INTRODUCTION

Patients presenting for thoracic surgery often have lung or bronchial carcinoma, a mediastinal mass, or esophageal disease. They typically are elderly, with a history of smoking and consequent comorbid conditions. The preoperative evaluation is an assessment of cardiac and pulmonary function with an aim to optimize these patients for a surgical procedure. Optimization may be limited, however, due to the underlying surgical disease. Ultimately, the decision to perform an operation or not depends on the risk of perioperative morbidity and also the predicted quality of life after surgery. Preoperative evaluation and testing aim to identify those patients who will tolerate a surgical intervention.

PHYSIOLOGIC EFFECTS OF CHEST SURGERY

The position on the operating room table effects a patient's underlying cardiopulmonary physiology. Thoracic surgery typically is performed in the lateral decubitus position with the operative side up. Additional physiologic changes occur when the chest cavity is opened. Likewise, optimal surgical exposure often requires collapse of the operative lung, creating further physiologic challenges.

All these changes must be considered when making a decision on whether or not a patient will tolerate thoracic surgery.

Lateral Decubitus Position/Closed Chest

Perfusion (Q) of the nonoperative lung is greater than the operative lung because of the effects of gravity on the pulmonary circulation. The converse applies for the distribution of ventilation (V) between the lungs during invasive positive pressure ventilation. The resultant changes in ventilation and perfusion cause V/Q mismatch and shunt. The operative lung is well ventilated and poorly perfused, causing V/Q mismatch. Subsequently, the nonoperative lung is poorly ventilated and well perfused, leading to shunt. Additional challenges and further V/Q mismatch present when the operative lung is collapsed intraoperatively.

Lateral Decubitus Position/Open Chest

When the chest wall is open, compliance of the operative lung increases because it is less restricted by the chest wall. The increased compliance leads to further increases in the amount of ventilation directed to the operative lung and away from the nonoperative lung, which can lead

[a] Division of Critical Care Medicine, Department of Anesthesiology and Perioperative Medicine, University of Massachusetts Medical School, UMass Memorial Medical Center, 55 Lake Avenue North, Worcester, MA 01655, USA; [b] Department of Anesthesiology, Division of Critical Care, UMass Memorial Medical Center, Worcester, MA, USA; [c] Boston University School of Medicine, Boston, MA, USA
* Corresponding author.
E-mail addresses: Theofilos.matheos2@umassmemorial.org; Theofilos.matheos@gmail.com

Thorac Surg Clin 30 (2020) 241–247
https://doi.org/10.1016/j.thorsurg.2020.04.003
1547-4127/20/© 2020 Elsevier Inc. All rights reserved.

to worsening V/Q mismatch. Under normal circumstances, the distribution of perfusion is not greatly affected by the opening of the chest. If there is a large increase in the compliance and subsequent decrease in airway pressure of the operative lung, however, perfusion to the operative lung may increase, improving shunt.

One Lung Ventilation

When ventilation to the operative lung ceases, an obligatory shunt of 20% to 30% is created, because perfusion to the operative lung persists. This leads to a reduction in Pao_2. The major determinants of blood flow to the operative lung include gravity, underlying lung disease, surgical interference including clamping of the pulmonary artery, and hypoxic pulmonary vasoconstriction (HPV).

In the nonoperative lung, blood flow is determined by gravity, underlying lung disease, ventilation strategies, and HPV. The mode of ventilation is an important consideration; a reduction in tidal volume during 1 lung ventilation can result in atelectasis and increased shunt. Hyperventilation of the nonoperative lung may inhibit HPV, resulting in blood diversion to poorly oxygenated areas. Excessively high airway pressures result in an increase in pulmonary vascular resistance of the ventilated lung, leading to diversion of blood to the nonventilated lung.

Hypoxic Pulmonary Vasoconstriction

HPV maintains arterial oxygenation by diverting blood flow away from poorly ventilated areas of lung. Typically, this occurs in areas of atelectasis or low V/Q ratio. HPV may be inhibited by vasodilatory medications, such as nitroprusside, nitroglycerine, calcium channel blockers, and β_2-agonists. The HPV response is maximal at normal pulmonary artery pressures and decreases at both high and low pulmonary artery pressures. Both high and low Pvo_2 conditions inhibit HPV. A low Pvo_2 causes HPV to occur in normoxic alveoli, diverting flow away from those alveoli. This is why a reduction in cardiac output during 1 lung ventilation may result in severe hypoxemia. HPV also is inhibited by hypocapnia and enhanced by hypercapnia.

COMORBID CONDITIONS
Age

There is no upper age limit when considering lung resection surgery. Physiologic age is a better predictor of outcomes than chronologic age. Operative mortality rates related to surgical intervention in patients aged 80 years to 90 years are approximately 1.4% and long-term outcomes appear satisfactory; however, patient comorbidities and mediastinal lymph node dissection have been identified as factors that increase the risk of postoperative complications in this population.[1]

Cough

Cough can be suggestive of pulmonary or cardiac disease. Elevated pulmonary artery pressures leading to interstitial and alveolar edema indicate cardiac etiology. Cough with expectoration for months and years commonly occurs in chronic obstructive pulmonary disease (COPD) or bronchitis. Initial assessment must be tailored to recognize triggers, such as medications, environmental factors, smoking, and COPD. Infectious etiology must be considered.

Dyspnea

Dyspnea also is a common symptom of lung and cardiac disease. When dyspnea is combined with cough or sputum, it most often is due to pulmonary disease. Inspiratory dyspnea suggests obstruction of the upper airway whereas expiratory dyspnea is more indicative of lower airway obstruction. Paroxysmal nocturnal dyspnea develops due to interstitial and interalveolar edema.[2] If a cough develops before paroxysmal nocturnal dyspnea, it most likely is related to chronic pulmonary disease; however, if cough develops after symptoms of dyspnea, it likely is due to left ventricular failure.

Tobacco Use

Smoking status is a risk factor for developing several postoperative complications, including respiratory failure, intensive care unit admission, pneumonia, and wound infection, among others. Abstinence from cigarette smoking can improve perioperative outcomes and decrease the risk of cardiovascular and respiratory complications, although the necessary duration of abstinence to achieve this risk reduction is debated. Smoking cessation 12 hours to 48 hours prior to surgery reduces carboxyhemoglobin levels in the blood and shifts the oxyhemoglobin dissociation curve to increase oxygen-carrying capacity. Smoking cessation for approximately 2 weeks improves ciliary function and reduces bronchial secretions. Cessation for 4 weeks to 8 weeks before surgery decreases postoperative pulmonary complications considerably. The benefits of nicotine replacement therapies in abstaining smokers seem to outweigh the risks of continued smoking.[3]

Chronic Obstructive Pulmonary Disease

COPD is the most common comorbid condition in patients presenting for thoracic surgery. It is characterized by a reduction in airflow that is not fully reversible. The severity of COPD is classified based on spirometry findings and correlates with an increasing risk of postoperative pulmonary complications as airflow limitation increases.[4] Patients with severe COPD often have concomitant right ventricular dysfunction and cor pulmonale. These patients pose unique challenges during intraoperative management, particularly during 1 lung ventilation for both surgeons and anesthesiologists.

Lung Cancer

Lung cancer is the leading cause of cancer death for both men and women in the United States.[5] Resectability of the cancer refers to whether or not a tumor can be resected completely based on anatomic location. Operability takes into account the functional status of the patient and characterizes a patient's ability to tolerate the procedure.

Hypertension

Systemic hypertension is a known risk factor for postoperative cardiovascular complications. Preoperative evaluation should aim to rule out secondary causes for hypertension, such as renal artery stenosis and pheochromocytoma. It should evaluate the severity of the disease, which requires multiple blood pressure readings on separate occasions. It also should identify evidence of target organ involvement. Examples of target organ involvement may include coronary disease, cerebrovascular disease, impaired renal function, and signs of left ventricular hypertrophy or heart failure. Patients who have severe hypertension or moderate hypertension with target organ involvement should have their blood pressure controlled before surgery. Surgery should not be deferred, however, on the basis of a single elevated blood pressure reading in the preoperative period, except for grade 3 hypertension. A patient's antihypertensive medications should be continued during the perioperative period, with the exception of angiotensin-converting enzyme inhibitors and angiotensin receptor blockers, which can cause profound and prolonged systemic hypotension during general anesthesia.[6,7]

Diabetes Mellitus

Diabetes mellitus has an impact on multiple organ systems. The disease presents increased risks for perioperative complications including myocardial infarction, stroke, limb ischemia, pressure sores, wound infection, and more. Preoperative evaluation should assess compliance with medications and symptoms of autonomic dysfunction. Blood glucose levels should be within normal limits before surgery. It is typical to discontinue long-acting oral hypoglycemic agents on the day of surgery yet continue insulin regimens the evening before. Type 1 diabetics mellitus should have basal insulin pumps continued to prevent diabetic ketoacidosis.[8]

PREOPERATIVE ASSESSMENT
Airway Assessment

Airway assessment is an essential part of the preoperative evaluation of any surgical patient. The aim is to predict potential difficulties with mask ventilation and endotracheal intubation based on a patient's physical features and to develop a management plan accordingly. This is important especially for placement of double-lumen endotracheal tubes, which technically can be more challenging than single-lumen tubes. Anatomic features with airway implications include Mallampati score, ability to open the mouth, thyromental distance, neck mobility, and neck circumference.

Lung Examination

Respiratory rate, regularity, and depth and effort of breathing should be observed. Restrictive lung disease is characterized by rapid shallow respirations, whereas obstructive disease features slow deep respirations. Asymmetric chest movement can occur due to phrenic nerve pathology, pneumothorax, or pleural effusion. On percussion, hyperresonance is indicative of emphysema or pneumothorax. Dullness suggests pleural effusion, atelectasis, or pneumonia. On auscultation of the lungs, prolonged expiration, expiratory wheezes, and rhonchi are indicative of obstructive lung disease. Absent breath sounds may indicate pleural effusion or atelectasis. Bronchial breath sounds are suggestive of pneumonia.

CARDIAC RISK STRATIFICATION

The revised cardiac risk index (RCRI) is used to predict the chances of a patient developing major cardiac complications after noncardiac surgery. A modified RCRI has been developed and validated to predict this risk in patients specifically after lung resection. The 4 items included in the recalibrated RCRI are cerebrovascular disease, cardiac ischemia, renal disease, and pneumonectomy. The screening tool can be used for cardiac risk stratification prior to thoracic surgery and for selecting those patients who may benefit from preoperative cardiology consultation and further cardiac testing.[9,10]

LABORATORY AND IMAGING STUDIES
Complete Blood Cell Count and Metabolic Studies

Complete blood cell count may reveal polycythemia caused by chronic tobacco use. Liver function tests may be abnormal due to metastatic lung cancer. Elevations in calcium may be due to bone metastasis or a paraneoplastic syndrome associated with tumor. Syndrome of inappropriate antidiuretic hormone may occur in squamous cell lung cancer and may cause hyponatremia. Elevated alkaline phosphatase may be a result of liver or bone metastasis.

Chest Radiography

A baseline chest radiograph often is included in the assessment of patients presenting for thoracic surgery. Important radiographic findings with perioperative implications include tracheal deviation or obstruction, pleural effusion implying diminished vital capacity and functional residual capacity, bullous lung disease at risk of rupture from positive pressure ventilation, cavitation with air fluid levels suggesting infectious process, and alveolar or interstitial infiltrates that contribute to V/Q mismatch and shunt.

Chest Computed Tomography

It is routine for lung cancer patients to have a computed tomography (CT) scan of the chest to determine anatomy of the tumor, nodal involvement, and metastatic spread. Thus, CT scan has a role in evaluation and staging of lung cancer, helping to decide on management strategy and operative approach. The limitation of CT scan is the reduced precision for recognizing mediastinal lymph node metastasis compared with PET-CT scan.[11]

Electrocardiogram

The simplicity of electrocardiogram and its capability to provide details of the electrical functions of the heart makes it important in assessment of patients with cardiothoracic pathology. New-onset arrhythmias, such as atrial fibrillation or left bundle branch block, should be investigated further prior to surgery. Evidence of left ventricular hypertrophy in a patient with systemic hypertension may indicate target organ involvement and necessitate preoperative blood pressure optimization.

Arterial Blood Gas

Arterial blood gas analysis can be performed on patients who are considered for lung resection, although this test is not required preoperatively.[12] Baseline oxygenation and ventilation values can aid in intraoperative ventilator management and postoperative care of the thoracic surgery patient; however, arterial P_{O_2} and P_{CO_2} have not been shown to predict postoperative complication rates accurately.

PULMONARY FUNCTION TESTING

Surgical resection often is the only curative option for non–small cell lung cancer; however, many of these patients have limited pulmonary reserve. Resection of functional lung tissue may result in an unacceptably poor quality of life after recovery from surgery. The underlying purpose of preoperative pulmonary function testing is to predict the functional status and quality of life of these patients after surgery as well as the risk of postoperative morbidity.

Spirometry

Measured forced expiratory volume in 1 second (FEV_1) is an essential assessment tool when evaluating a patient for thoracic surgery. FEV_1 predicts the degree of respiratory impairment in patients with COPD. Patients with a preoperative FEV_1 greater than 80% predicted often can tolerate pneumonectomy and with greater than 70% predicted can tolerate lobectomy. A preoperative FEV_1 less than 60% predicted is a strong indicator of postoperative respiratory complications and 30-day mortality.[13]

Diffusing capacity of carbon monoxide (DLCO) can determine the presence of emphysematous changes in lung tissue. Preoperative DLCO has been shown to significantly predict mortality and postoperative pulmonary complications after lung resection. DLCO values less than 60% are considered inappropriate for major lung resections whereas DLCO greater than 70% is associated with decreased postoperative complication rates.[14]

Predicted Postoperative Lung Function

Predicted postoperative (PPO) lung function studies determine the contribution of the segment of the lung to be resected to a patient's overall lung function, thereby allowing for a prediction of the patient's postoperative pulmonary function status.

These studies were first described in the 1970s and are used routinely today.[15] Quantitative radionuclide perfusion lung scanning is recommended to determine PPO FEV_1 and PPO DLCO for patients requiring pneumonectomy. In patients undergoing lobectomy, however, the anatomic method of segmental counting can be used.[16]

PPO FEV_1 and PPO DLCO should be calculated in all patients whose baseline FEV_1 and DLCO are less than 80% predicted. PPO FEV_1 and PPO DLCO values greater than 60% indicate low risk of postoperative morbidity after major anatomic lung resection. PPO FEV_1 and PPO DLCO values between 30% and 60% warrant a low-technology exercise test, such as stair climbing or 6-minute walk tests.[17] The stair climbing test has been shown an adequate predictor of postoperative pulmonary and cardiac complications and is both safe and economical; however, standardizing the test has been challenging.[18]

Cardiopulmonary Exercise Testing

Cardiopulmonary exercise testing (CPET) is used to evaluate for abnormalities in oxygen transport that may be masked at rest. CPET calculates maximal oxygen consumption (Vo_{2max}), an indicator of cardiorespiratory fitness, which can be used to predict a patient's ability to tolerate certain thoracic surgical procedures. CPET is indicated when either the calculated PPO FEV_1 or PPO DLCO is less than 30% predicted. A Vo_{2max} greater than 20 mL/kg/min is preferred for patients undergoing pneumonectomy whereas Vo_2max greater than 15 mL/kg/min may be acceptable for lobectomy. Vo_{2max} less than 10 mL/kg/min indicates a high risk of mortality after major anatomic lung resection and necessitates the calculation of PPO Vo_{2max}.[17]

THE PREOPERATIVE VISIT

The stress of surgery induces a catabolic state that leads to increased cardiac demand, relative tissue hypoxia, increased insulin resistance, impaired coagulation profiles, and altered pulmonary and gastrointestinal function. This response can lead to organ dysfunction, increased morbidity, and delayed surgical recovery.[19] Colorectal surgery was the first surgical subspecialty to conceptualize the idea of enhanced recovery after surgery (ERAS). Some of the benefits of ERAS programs include reductions in hospital length of stay, decreased postoperative complication rates without changes in readmission rates,[20] and improved patient satisfaction.[21] Enhanced recovery after thoracic surgery (ERATS) programs

have since been created with similar principles in mind.[22]

The term, ERATS, implies an emphasis on care after surgery; however, the process begins in the preoperative period, well before a patient's surgery. This is the time to engage patients, educate them on the steps of their journey, and manage their expectations. It is the time to task patients with taking an active part in their care, from preparation to recovery. This also is the time to optimize patients, both physically and mentally. Prescribed fitness regimens,[23] nutritional support, and smoking cessation counseling[24] all can improve baseline functional status and contribute to better postoperative outcomes.

Optimized medication regimens, especially for patients with known or newly diagnosed COPD, is a key component to improving postoperative outcomes. Pulmonary status optimization requires close review of prescribed medications, symptoms, and pulmonary function so that medications can be adjusted to be consistent with the current guidelines.[25] Even marginal gains in preoperative FEV_1 can have perioperative benefits. When COPD is a new diagnosis, there is evidence to suggest that short-term benefits can be made on FEV_1 and COPD severity within 1 week of initiating new therapies.[26]

Traditional fasting requirements the night before surgery deplete liver glycogen and are associated with impaired glucose metabolism and increased insulin resistance. Data from the anesthesia literature have demonstrated that intake of clear fluids up until 2 hours before surgery does not increase gastric content volume, reduce gastric fluid pH, or increase complication rates. Thus, in contrast to traditional nil per os strategies, clear liquids, including oral carbohydrate drinks, should be allowed up to 2 hours before induction of anesthesia and light meals up to 6 hours prior.[27] This can avoid dehydration, reduce preoperative thirst and anxiety, and reduce postoperative interleukin-6 levels and insulin resistance, all of which have a positive impact on hospital length of stay and patient satisfaction.[28,29]

SUMMARY

Preoperative assessment is the critical first step for all patients considered for thoracic surgery. It is the time when surgeons decide if a patient is a surgical candidate or not. For those individuals deemed surgical candidates, it is the time for them to become educated on their perioperative course so that realistic expectations can be set. Most critically, it is the time for surgical candidates to improve their chances at survival and reduce their risk of morbidity with a prescribed optimization regimen. Successful outcomes and mitigated surgical risk start with the preoperative evaluation.

DISCLOSURE

The authors have nothing to disclose.

REFERENCES

1. Okami J, Higashiyama M, Asamura H, et al. Pulmonary resection in patients aged 80 years or over with clinical stage I non-small cell lung cancer: prognostic factors for overall survival and risk factors for postoperative complications. J Thorac Oncol 2009;4(10):1247–53.
2. Braunwald E. Examination of the patient: the history. In: Braunwald E, editor. Heart disease: a textbook of cardiovascular medicine. 5th edition. Philadelphia: Saunders; 1997. p. p1.
3. Warner DO. Perioperative abstinence from cigarettes: physiologic and clinical consequences. Anesthesiology 2006;104(2):356–67.
4. Shin B, Le H, Kang D, et al. Airflow limitation severity and post-operative pulmonary complications following extra-pulmonary surgery in COPD patients. Respirology 2017;22(5):935–41.
5. Lung cancer statistics. Centers for Disease Control and Preventon. 2019. Available at: https://www.cdc.gov/cancer/lung/statistics/. Accessed March 25, 2020.
6. Foex P, Sear JW. The surgical hypertensive patient. Continuing Educ Anaesth Crit Care Pain 2004;4(5):169–71.
7. Lapage KG, Wouters PF. The patient with hypertension undergoing surgery. Curr Opin Anaesthesiol 2016;29(3):397–402.
8. Schmiesing CA, Brodsky JB. The preoperative anesthesia evaluation. Thorac Surg Clin 2005;15(2):305–15.
9. Brunelli A, Varela G, Salati M, et al. Recalibration of the revised cardiac risk index in lung resection candidates. Ann Thorac Surg 2010;90(1):199–203.
10. Ferguson MK, Celauro AD, Vigneswaran WT. Validation of a modified scoring system for cardiovascular risk associated with major lung resection. Eur J Cardiothorasic Surg 2012;41(3):598–602.
11. Silvestri GA, Gonzalez AV, Jantz MA, et al. Methods of staging non-small cell lung cancer: diagnosis and management of lung cancer, 3rd ed: American College of Chest Physicians evidence based clinical practice guidelines. Chest 2013;143(5 Suppl):e211S–50s.
12. Dunn WF, Scanlon PD. Preoperative pulmonary function testing for patients with lung cancer. Mayo Clin Proc 1993;68:371.
13. Licker MJ, Widikker I, Robert J, et al. Operative mortality and respiratory complications after lung resection for cancer impact of chronic obstructive pulmonary disease and time trends. Ann Thorac Surg 2006;81(5):1830–7.
14. Ferguson MK, Little L, Rizzo L, et al. Diffusing capacity predicts morbidity and mortality after pulmonary resection. J Thorac Cardiovasc Surg 1998;96:894–900.
15. Tonnesen KG, Dige-Petersen H, Lund JO, et al. Lung split function test and pneumonectomy. A lower limit for operability. Scand J Thorac Cardiovasc Surg 1978;12(2):133–6.
16. British Thoracic Society. BTS guidelines: guidelines on the selection of patients with lung cancer for surgery. Thorax 2001;56(2):89–108.
17. Brunelli A, Kim AW, Berger KI, et al. Physiologic evaluation of the patient with lung cancer being considered for resection surgery. Chest 2013;143(5 Suppl):e166s–90s.
18. Brunelli A, Refai M, Monteverde M, et al. Stair climbing test predicts cardiopulmonary complications after lung resection. Chest 2002;121(4):1106–10.
19. Wilmore DW. From Cuthbertson to fast-track surgery: 70 years of progress in reducing stress in surgical patients. Ann Surg 2002;236(5):643–8.
20. Varadhan KK, Neal KR, Dejong CH, et al. The enhanced recovery after surgery (ERAS) pathway for patients undergoing major elective open colorectal surgery: a meta-analysis of randomized controlled trials. Clin Nutr 2010;29(4):434–40.
21. Philp S, Carter J, Pather S, et al. Patients' satisfaction with fast-track surgery in gynaecological oncology. Eur J Cancer Care (Engl) 2015;24:567–73.
22. Scarci M, Solli P, Bedetti B. Enhanced recovery pathway for thoracic surgery in the UK. J Thorac Dis 2016;8(Suppl 1):S78–83.
23. Pouwels S, Fiddelaers J, Teijink JA, et al. Preoperative exercise therapy in lung surgery patients: a systematic review. Respir Med 2015;109(12):1495–504.
24. Mason DP, Subramanian S, Nowicki ER, et al. Impact of smoking cessation before resection of lung cancer: a Society of Thoracic Surgeons General Thoracic Surgery Database study. Ann Thorac Surg 2009;88(2):362–70.
25. Qaseem A, Wilt TJ, Weinberger SE, et al. Diagnosis and management of stable chronic obstructive pulmonary disease: a clinical practice guideline update from the American College of Physicians, American College of Chest Physicians, American Thoracic Society, and European Respiratory Society. Ann Intern Med 2011;155(3):179–91.
26. Bolukbas S, Eberlein M, Eckhoff J, et al. Short-term effects of inhalative tiotropium/formoterol/budesonide versus tiotropium/formoterol in patients with newly diagnosed chronic obstructive pulmonary

disease requiring surgery for lung cancer: a prospective randomized trial. Eur J Cardiothroac Surg 2011;39(6):995–1000.

27. Practice guidelines for preoperative fasting and the use of pharmacologic agents to reduce the risk of pulmonary aspiration: application to healthy patients undergoing elective procedures: an updated report by the American Society of Anesthesiologists Task Force on Preoperative Fasting and the Use of Pharmacologic Agents to Reduce the Risk of Pulmonary Aspiration. Anesthesiology 2017; 126(3):376–93.

28. Rizvanovic N, Nesek AV, Causevic S, et al. A randomised controlled study of preoperative oral carbohydrate loading versus fasting in patients undergoing colorectal surgery. Int J Colorectal Dis 2019;34(9):1551–61.

29. Noblett SE, Watson DS, Huong H, et al. Pre-operative oral carbohydrate loading in colorectal surgery: a randomized controlled trial. Colorectal Dis 2006;8:563–9.

Prehabilitation of the Thoracic Surgery Patient

Aaron R. Dezube, MD[a],[*],[1], Lisa Cooper, MD[b],[1], Michael T. Jaklitsch, MD[a]

KEYWORDS

• Older adults • Thoracic surgery • Frailty • Prehabilitation

KEY POINTS

- Physiologic age rather than chronologic age is a better predictor of outcomes after thoracic surgery.
- Useful assessment tools exist to identify frailty in older patients, such as clinical frailty scales, frailty index, frail screening scale, and frailty phenotype, which may identify appropriate candidates for prehabilitation. Assessment is done best in a multidisciplinary fashion between primary care, geriatricians, and thoracic surgeons.
- Preoperative exercise-based intervention (prehabilitation) has demonstrated reduction of morbidity and mortality in other surgeries but in thoracic surgery continues to be under discussion with heterogeneous but potentially promising results.

INTRODUCTION

In thoracic surgery the 2 main groups of high-risk patients are young adults with comorbidities, mainly chronic lung and heart disease, and older adults, mainly with frailty. This review focuses on these 2 different populations and on strategies to define and better prepare them for surgery and thus improve postoperative outcomes.

Many older patients, defined as those patients 65 years or older, present an array of challenges when undergoing thoracic surgery. Although advances in minimally invasive techniques have made it feasible for the older population to undergo thoracic surgery safely,[1],[2] elderly patients are more likely to have complications,[3] have longer lengths of stay,[2],[4] and are more likely to require involved discharge planning, including need for home health aides or formal rehabilitation.[5]

Preoperative rehabilitation (prehabilitation) can optimize functional and nutritional capacity and serve as a teachable moment in which healthy lifestyle changes actively can be made.[6] Prehabilitation has 2 parts: (1) the identification of preoperative conditions that are associated with postoperative morbidity and (2) an attempt to minimize these conditions preoperatively with the hope it will result in better outcomes. Furthermore, when looking at mortality after elective surgery, it frequently is characterized by multiorgan dysfunction. In fact, 1 study compared major surgery to running a marathon. Few adults can go out and run a marathon without training, but, after several months of regular training, some could complete this goal.[6] Their bodies did not grow additional heart and lung tissue, but their organs became more efficient. This analogy is an attractive comparison, particularly to prehabilitation, because marathon training also has developed its own science. Prehabilitation tries to improve multiple organ systems prior to elective surgery.

[a] Division of Thoracic Surgery, Brigham and Women's Hospital, 75 Francis Street, Boston, MA 02115, USA;
[b] Division of Aging, Brigham and Women's Hospital, 75 Francis Street, Boston, MA 02115, USA
[1] Co-first author.
* Corresponding author.
E-mail address: adezube@partners.org

Thorac Surg Clin 30 (2020) 249–258
https://doi.org/10.1016/j.thorsurg.2020.04.004
1547-4127/20/© 2020 Elsevier Inc. All rights reserved.

History of Prehabilitation

Prehabilitation does not appear as a topic in the surgical textbooks of the 1980s. At that time, preoperative preparation for patients referred to immediate correction of blood volume, intravascular fluids, and electrolyte balance. There were no large databases. The under-appreciated personal computers became available in the 1990s. Surgical outcome reports were based on laborious chart reviews, usually from single institutions, and were prone to subtle selection biases of the lead surgeon. For elective cases, selection of patients was binary: either a patient was surgical candidate or not.

The Goldman criteria were published in 1977.[7] This was a landmark prospective study of preoperative variables that predicted cardiac events after major noncardiac surgery in 1001 patients over age 40. Data were collected from Massachusetts General Hospital from October 1975 to April 1976. By multivariate discriminant analysis, the investigators were able to identify 9 predictors: preoperative third heart sound or jugular venous distention; myocardial infarction in the preceding 6 months; more than 5 premature ventricular contractions per minute before operation; rhythm other than sinus or premature atrial contractions on preoperative electrocardiogram; age over 70 years; intraperitoneal, intrathoracic or aortic operation; emergency operation; important valvular aortic stenosis; and poor general medical condition. Patients could be separated into 4 classes of significantly different risk. Ten of the 19 postoperative cardiac fatalities occurred in the 18 patients at highest risk. The investigators created a clinical prediction rule. Of the maximum 53 possible points, 23 were potentially controllable.[8] The Goldman criteria became popular as a method to identify elevated risk for elective surgery and a way to reduce that risk with preoperative intervention or timing.

The gold standards to judge the success of an operation have been the 30-day mortality rate and the disease recurrence rate. With modern critical care, a low 30-day mortality rate may be a reflection of an advanced intensive care unit team. Today, it is recognized that the 90-day mortality frequently is much higher than the 30-day mortality.[9] Even more ominous, a recent analysis shows that nursing home placement 1 year after surgery is a function of age.[10] This is a poor outcome that was not measured 4 decades ago. Additionally, surgery for lung cancer can trigger a loss of independence that patients may deem unacceptable.[10,11]

Neoadjuvant chemoradiation trials for esophageal[12] and stage IIIA (N2) lung cancer[13,14] in the mid-1990s demonstrated to thoracic surgeons that dramatic but temporary declines in functional status might follow the neoadjuvant stage. The toxicity of combined chemoradiation frequently reduces the performance status of the patient temporarily. For some patients for whom the hope was to perform the surgical resection by 4 weeks after the neoadjuvant therapy, their frailty interfered with the plan. On later reassessment, the clinicians found that these same frail patients had improved their strength and functional status with an additional 2 weeks to 6 weeks of recovery time, thus making them strong enough for an operation. This experience taught a generation of thoracic surgeons that performance status could be improved prior to surgery.

Identification of Candidates for Prehabilitation

Often frailty is the metric utilized to identify those who may benefit from prehabilitation. Frailty is a syndrome of decreased reserve and resistance to stressors resulting from cumulative declines across multiple physiologic systems and causing vulnerability to adverse outcomes.[15] Frailty, although more prevalent in older adults, is not limited to this population[16,17] and is important to recognize and quantify. The presence of frailty and degree of severity are known to be predictors of worse postoperative outcomes.[18,19] Therefore, it remains critical to identify high-risk surgical candidates and target modifiable risk factors (pulmonary and cardiac function; functional capacity; degree of lung resection; cognitive reserve and delirium risk; polypharmacy; and nutritional status) to improve postoperative outcomes.

It is accepted that operative risk is associated more closely with functional status, frailty, and physiologic age rather than chronologic age.[20–22] High rates of frailty have been identified on a national level as present in 15.3% of patients greater than 65 years old, with notable variation by region, race/ethnicity, and income.[23] In thoracic surgery, preoperative patients appear to have even higher rates, with estimate prevalence of frailty and prefrailty as high as 68.8% of older patients.[24]

The thoracic surgery patient routinely suffers from multiple comorbidities in addition to higher rates of frailty. These may have an impact on their surgical outcomes. Outcomes also may be impacted by higher rates of chronic obstructive pulmonary disease (COPD) and decreased pulmonary reserve, including physiologic changes of the respiratory system. These changes include but are not limited to reduced chest wall compliance, reduction of elastic recoil, and decreased alveolar gas exchange, resulting in decreased P_{O_2} and forced expiratory volume in the first second of expiration (FEV_1). In addition, there are higher rates of malnutrition and sarcopenia in esophageal cancer patients related to their prevalence of smoking and ethanol use. All these factors are associated with worse postoperative morbidity and mortality in thoracic surgery.[25,26]

Assessment of frailty in addition to routine preoperative work-up includes validated metrics, such as clinical frailty scale (**Fig. 1**),[27] frailty phenotype, and the more detailed frailty index.[15,28–31] Higher frailty index has been associated with increased 30-day complications, failure to wean from ventilator, reintubation, surgical site infection, pneumonia, and grade 4 complications after lobectomy.[32,33] These tools are important in identifying frail older adults, thus introducing an opportunity to increase functional and nutritional reserves to decrease the decline in the postoperative period.[6]

In addition to traditional preoperative work-up, consisting of laboratory tests, and imaging such as echocardiogram or stress tests, high-risk patients may be identified with frailty scales, geriatric assessment, performance of physical examination, and physiologic testing. Physical examination should be directed for signs of COPD, pulmonary hypertension, arthritis, kyphosis, and hiatal hernias. Standard physiologic tests include pulmonary function testing, 6-minute walk tests (6MWTs), and exercise-induced hypoxia testing. Absolute step count recently has been noted to be not predictive of postoperative outcome.[34] These previously listed assessment practices are aligned with the recently published recommendations from the American College of Surgeons and the American Geriatrics Society.[35] At minimum, the team should evaluate in the preoperative period the following domains to identify high-risk vulnerable patients: those with impaired cognition, delirium risk, impaired functional status, impaired mobility, malnutrition, difficulty swallowing, and in need of a palliative care assessment. Ways to assess and address frailty as well as screen for cognitive impairment (eg, mini-cognitive test) among older adults who are candidates for surgical interventions have been published by the Society of Perioperative Assessment and Quality Improvement and include the different methods available and how to best utilize them in the perioperative period (**Fig. 2**).[36,37]

Modern-day Evidence for Prehabilitation

Use of prehabilitation originated outside of thoracic surgery. In cardiac surgery, prehabilitation was shown to reduce hospital length of stay.[38] After major abdominal surgery, patients who underwent formal prehabilitation prior to colectomy had fewer complications and an average savings of $21,946 per patient.[39] This

Clinical Frailty Scale*

 1 Very Fit – People who are robust, active, energetic and motivated. These people commonly exercise regularly. They are among the fittest for their age.

 2 Well – People who have **no active disease** symptoms but are less fit than category 1. Often, they exercise or are very **active occasionally**, e.g. seasonally.

 3 Managing Well – People whose **medical problems are well controlled**, but are **not regularly active** beyond routine walking.

 4 Vulnerable – While **not dependent** on others for daily help, often **symptoms limit activities**. A common complaint is being "slowed up", and/or being tired during the day.

 5 Mildly Frail – These people often have **more evident slowing**, and need help in **high order IADLs** (finances, transportation, heavy housework, medications). Typically, mild frailty progressively impairs shopping and walking outside alone, meal preparation and housework.

 6 Moderately Frail – People need help with **all outside activities** and with **keeping house**. Inside, they often have problems with stairs and need **help with bathing** and might need minimal assistance (cuing, standby) with dressing.

 7 Severely Frail – **Completely dependent** for personal care, from whatever cause (physical or cognitive). Even so, they seem stable and not at high risk of dying (within ~ 6 mo).

8 Very Severely Frail – Completely dependent, approaching the end of life. Typically, they could not recover even from a minor illness.

 9 Terminally Ill - Approaching the end of life. This category applies to people with a life expectancy <6 mo, who are **not otherwise evidently frail**.

Scoring frailty in people with dementia

The degree of frailty corresponds to the degree of dementia. Common symptoms in mild dementia include forgetting the details of a recent event, though still remembering the event itself, repeating the same question/story and social withdrawal.

In moderate dementia, recent memory is very impaired, even though they seemingly can remember their past life events well. They can do personal care with prompting.

In severe dementia, they cannot do personal care without help.

* 1. Canadian Study on Health & Aging, Revised 2008.
2. K. Rockwood et al. A global clinical measure of fitness and frailty in elderly people. CMAJ 2005;173:489-495.

Fig. 1. Clinical frailty scale. (*From* Rockwood K, Song X, MacKnight C, et al. A global clinical measure of fitness and frailty in elderly people. CMAJ 2005;173(5):489–95. ©2007-2009 Version 1.2. Canadian Study on health and Aging Revision 2008.)

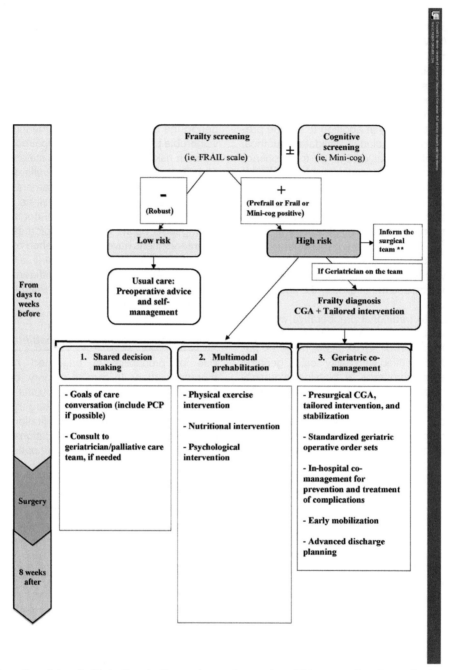

Fig. 2. Operationalizing frailty in the elective perioperative setting. CGA, comprehensive geriatric assessment; PCP, primary care physician. (*From* Alvarez-Nebreda ML, Bentov N, Urman RD, et al. Recommendations for preoperative management of frailty from the Society for Perioperative Assessment and Quality Improvement (SPAQI). J Clin Anesth 2018;47:37; with permission.)

has been similarly validated for pulmonary rehabilitation and inspiratory muscle training to prevent atelectasis. For example, after cardiac surgery, in a single-blind randomized trial by Hulzebos and colleagues,[40] those who underwent preoperative inspiratory muscle training had reduced odds of postoperative pulmonary complications (odds ratio [OR] 0.52; 95% CI, 0.30–0.92), pneumonia (OR 0.40%; 95% CI, 0.19–0.84), and shorter length of stay (LOS) (median 7 days vs 8 days, respectively; $P = .02$). No outcome change, however, was shown for simple preoperative information

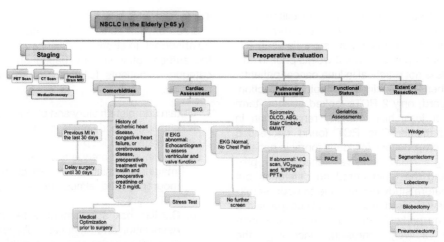

Fig. 3. Proposed algorithm work-up of NSCLC in the elderly patient. ABG, arterial blood gas; BGA, blood gas analysis; CT, computed tomography; EKG, electrocardiogram; MI, myocardial infarction; MRI, magnetic resonance imaging; NSCLC, non–small cell lung cancer; PACE, preoperative assessment of cancer in elderly; PPO, predicted postoperative; V/Q, ventilation/perfusion. (*From* Bravo-Iñiguez C, Perez Martinez M, Armstrong KW, et al. Surgical resection of lung cancer in the elderly. Thorac Surg Clin 2014;24(4):378; with permission.)

booklet and diaries without physical intervention.[41]

Within the realm of thoracic surgery, data and randomized controlled trials (RCTs) are more limited, with only circumstantial benefit in thoracic patients.[42–44]

In patients undergoing lung resection for lung cancer, the few RCTs that exist[45–48] had small sample sizes, with heterogeneous interventions ranging from strength training to inspiratory muscle training. One RCT looked at a multimodal prehabilitation program on perioperative functional capacity in patients undergoing video-assisted thoracoscopic surgery (VATS) lobectomy for non–small cell lung cancer. Their study found that a 14-day intervention increased the preoperative 6MWT and postoperative forced vital capacity (FVC) but did not show an improvement in clinical outcomes, such as LOS and complications.[49] Another study showed only circumstantial benefit in thoracic patients (weak recommendation), noting in their review that most previous studies lacked statistical power to demonstrate an effect on postoperative complication for thoracic surgery.[43] A recent systematic review of lung resection showed, however, intervention-based improvement in walking endurance, peak exercise capacity, dyspnea, risk of hospitalization, and postoperative pulmonary complications when there was a minimum of 1 week to 4 weeks with 1 session to 3 sessions per week at moderate intensity (50% of endurance capacity).[50] Pulmonary rehabilitation is recommended by professional societies for high-risk patients.[51–53] Finally, most prior studies on prehabilitation largely looked at older patients or frail patients. There is, however, limited evidence to suggest younger patients may achieve similar benefits from pulmonary rehabilitation.[54]

In esophageal cancer there is an even higher burden of care due to neoadjuvant chemoradiation in most cases followed by esophagectomy (a highly morbid procedure in many cases).[55,56] There also is a high prevalence of declined nutritional status due to the nature of this disease with weeks of dysphagia. On the other hand, this conveys a unique opportunity to prepare patients, especially older adults, for this complicated procedure. Prehabilitation that includes exercise and nutritional intervention was shown in 1 recent RCT[57] to improve functional capacity (study primary endpoints included walk distance, 6MWT, and proportion of patients who experienced a change in functional capacity) before and after esophagectomy. The RCT unfortunately was not powered enough to show any differences in their secondary outcomes (number and severity of complications, length of hospital stay, and readmission rates). In another study on prehabilitation by Soares and colleagues,[58] pulmonary function and physical performance were improved before and after upper abdominal surgery. Although there are some data showing that prehabilitation can improve outcomes in esophageal cancer, the overall benefits, including postoperative complications and oncology outcomes, are yet to be determined and remain an active area of research.[59]

Another issue surrounding prehabilitation of thoracic surgery relates to the time commitment. Although in other fields, such as cardiac surgery, it may be appropriate to wait 6 weeks prior to surgery,[60] this is not practical in lung cancer patients, who may benefit from timelier oncologic resection. In this regard, only 2 RCTs looked at short-term (1 week or less) high-intensity rehabilitation in thoracic patients. One RCT found decreased LOS and complications in elderly thoracic patients undergoing a 7-day intensive prehabilitation program,[61] and the other noted no difference but with premature study closure due to poor recruitment.[48] New RCTs in other surgical subspecialties investigating prehabilitation or exercise intervention are actively enrolling, including the PERFORM-TAVR study (NCT03522454),[62] the PREHAB study (NCT02219815),[63] and the PREQUEL trial.[60] The authors have identified no new RCTs in thoracic surgery, however, to investigate physical interventions, although there has been new interest in possible use of pedometer tracking as a possible tool.

Practice Recommendations

The authors' practice has synthesized the data, discussed previously, and developed their own best practice recommendations. The first step in their practice is to identify nonmodifiable variables (age, gender, stage, and family history) and, more importantly, modifiable variables (pulmonary and cardiac function, exercise capacity, amount of lung to be removed, polypharmacy, nutrition, and sleep) in a multidisciplinary office visit in conjunction with a geriatrician in older candidates. The steps in the authors' preoperative evaluation are listed. A flowchart for the work-up (see **Fig. 3**) and the authors' previously published minimum requirement functional cutoffs to consider candidacy for lung resection by degree of resection in older patients from their practice are provided in

Table 1,[64] which includes adjunct tests cutoffs, such as oxygen consumption, should initial tests be abnormal, to stratify surgical candidacy better; the authors offer surgery based on the lowest category a patients falls into based on cutoffs provided.

1. Obtain complete history and physical examination, including body mass index
2. Preoperative work-up
   a. Obtain basic preoperative laboratory tests, imaging (at minimum, chest computed tomography and almost universal use of a PET scan).
   b. Cardiac risk assessment (American Heart Association and American College of Cardiology)[65] provides easily accessible practice guidelines for need for electrocardiography, echocardiography, or stress test.
   c. Pulmonary assessment for lung resection patients includes pulmonary function tests (PFTs), including FEV_1, measurement of diffusing capacity of the lungs for carbon monoxide (DLCO), and room air arterial blood gas.
      i. Maximum oxygen consumption (Vo_{2max}), predicted postoperative lung function, and ventilation/perfusion scans may be used as adjuncts in setting of abnormal values to evaluate patients with marginal function.
3. In older patients, include comprehensive geriatric assessment.
   a. Use of clinical frailty scale (score 1–9), identification of frailty phenotype (prefrail if 1–2 factors met or frail if 3 or more criteria met, including unintentional weight loss, self-exhaustion, slow gait speed, low energy expenditure, and weak grip strength), or frailty index (individual deficits/number of measured deficits)

Table 1 Guidelines for lung resection in elderly patients			
Variables	**Lobectomy**	**Lesser Resection (Segment/Wedge)**	**Nonoperative Therapy**
Spirometry (FVC% or DLCO %PPO)	>50% PPO	25%–50% PPO	<25% PPO
6MWT (m)	400	60–400	<60 or wheelchair
Stair climbing (no. of flights)	2	<1	Unable to climb
Vo_{2max} (mL/kg/min)	>12	10–12	<10
Karnofsky Performance Status	70–100	30–60	<30

Abbreviation: PPO, predicted postoperative.
From Bravo-Iñiguez C, Perez Martinez M, Armstrong KW, et al. Surgical resection of lung cancer in the elderly. Thorac Surg Clin 2014;24(4):378; with permission.

b. Assess functional status, including activities of daily living and instruments of daily living

c. Performance status (Karnofsky Performance Status, Eastern Cooperative Oncology Group performance status)

d. Exercise tolerance tests: stair climbing, 6MWT, and most importantly walking distance

e. Measure of cognition and mood: Mini-Mental Status Examination, Geriatric Depression Scale, cognition and risk of postoperative confusion scale

f. Lifestyle adjustment

g. Social support: quality of life after surgery, new supports needed, possible loss of independence, and goals of care, including advance planning and code status

   i. Tobacco and alcohol abstinence for 7 days prior to surgery

   ii. Reduction in polypharmacy. Identify medications at risk of delirium (benzodiazepines and anticholinergics) and renal failure as well as develop β-blockade protocol, and discuss anticoagulation.

   iii. Sleep: recommend 6 hours to 8 hours of sleep per 24-hour period

   iv. Diet: calorie counts and quality of diet, possible nutrition laboratory tests

4. Prehabilitation

a. Recommend exercise 3 times a week for 1 hour. Reevaluate at 2-week mark if considering surgery with endpoints (kept appointment, exercised, and made objective improvement).

   i. Use this time to adjust nutrition, sleep, and mood.

   ii. Consider adjunct use of pedometers to measure walk distance.

5. Surgical planning and hospital course

a. Reassess surgical candidacy at regular intervals.

b. If having surgery, develop intrahospital plan (minimize high risk medication, develop sleep regimens, discuss postoperative fluid management, utilizie nonpharmacologic prevention and management of delirium, establish early recovery after surgery protcols and utilizie in-hospital geriatrician co-mangement or consultation).

Thoracic surgeons should be patient with pref-rail and frail patients, if the surgeons believe that prehabilitation has a role to play. The initial office visit should acknowledge the disease process and stage and the potential role of surgery. It should acknowledge which of the variables place the patient at risk. No decision in regard to surgery needs to be stated at this initial visit. Instead, an intervention plan should be laid out for the next 2 weeks. Patients and their family are instructed that in 2 weeks the team and the patient will meet again in a return office visit, and the spirometry and 6MWT or walk distance will be repeated.

In the authors' experience, there usually is 1 of 3 outcomes. The first possibility is that patients do not return to clinic, likely due to a realization that the physical tasks are beyond their capacity. The authors reach out to these patients and offer evaluation by a multidisciplinary team, including medical oncology, radiation oncology, and palliative care. The door remains open to this group should they seek reevaluation in the future. The second group returns with substantial improvement and frequently can make multiple milestones that indicate their risk of surgery has been substantially reduced. It is not known if this is a question of motivation, determination, or dramatic improvement in physical strength. Finally, the third group returns and are improved but have not yet reached the milestones that are associated with safe surgery. For these, the authors generally agree to continue the intervention program for an additional 2 weeks in the hope that there will be exponential improvement. If the prehabilitation is extending to 6 weeks, then the authors recommend that the multidisciplinary team, discussed previously, be consulted for alternative therapies. This method has proved successful in the authors' experience.

SUMMARY

Operative mortalities are at historic lows for nearly every major thoracic operation.[64] Even so, thoracic surgery patients tend to be older and have increased rates of frailty and other comorbidities, such as reduced pulmonary reserve, malnutrition, and sarcopenia, in additional to traditional comorbidities, such as cardiac-pulmonary disease, which are associated with worse surgical outcomes. Identification of physiologic reserve in the perioperative period should be performed in multidisciplinary collaboration with geriatricians as part of standardized work-up in the older adult (see **Fig. 2**). Targetable risk factors should be identified (pulmonary and cardiac function; exercise capacity; degree of lung resection; polypharmacy; nutrition; sleep; and lifestyle changes, including tobacco and alcohol cessation) and methods should be utilized to minimize these risk-factors in the preoperative setting and addressed with a well-planned, individualized prehabilitation program.

Prehabilitation has been validated as a tool to increase functional status of patients undergoing surgery in other specialties, and, although studies in thoracic surgery are more limited, with some heterogeneous outcomes, an overall trend to benefit has been observed. Although additional RCTs evaluating prehabilitation of thoracic surgery are required, the authors agree with professional societal recommendations to consider appropriate patients for prehabilitation if a nonemergent case is required. The authors believe screening of appropriate patients for prehabilitation services is the most likely method to further contribute to lower morbidity and mortality.

DISCLOSURE

The authors have nothing to disclose.

REFERENCES

1. Ryuichi S, Sadanori T, Motoharu H, et al. The perioperative complications for elderly patients with lung cancer associated with a pulmonary resection under general anesthesia. J Thorac Oncol 2009;4(2): 193–7.

2. Jaklitsch M, DeCamp M, Liptay M, et al. Video-assisted thoracic surgery in the elderly - A review of 307 cases. Chest 1996;110:751–8.

3. Darling Gail E, Allen Mark S, Decker Paul A, et al. Randomized trial of mediastinal lymph node sampling versus complete lymphadenectomy during pulmonary resection in the patient with N0 or N1 (less than hilar) non-small cell carcinoma: results of the American College of Surgery Oncology Group Z0030 Trial. J Thorac Cardiovasc Surg 2011; 141(3):662–70.

4. Giambrone Greg P, Smith Matthew C, Wu X, et al. Variability in length of stay after uncomplicated pulmonary lobectomy: is length of stay a quality metric or a patient metric? Eur J Cardiothorac Surg 2016; 49(4):e65–71.

5. Balentine Courtney J, Naik Aanand D, Berger David H, et al. Postacute care after major abdominal surgery in elderly patients: intersection of age, functional status, and postoperative complications. JAMA Surg 2016;151(8):759–66.

6. Prehabilitation: preparing patients for surgery. - PubMed - NCBI. Available at: https://www.ncbi.nlm. nih.gov/pubmed/28790033. Accessed March 27, 2020.

7. Goldman L, Caldera DL, Nussbaum SR, et al. Multifactorial index of cardiac risk in noncardiac surgical procedures. N Engl J Med 1977;297(16):845–50.

8. Brown Kristen N, Cascella M. Goldman risk indices. StatPearls. Treasure Island (FL): StatPearls Publishing; 2020.

9. White A, Kucukak S, Bueno R, et al. Pneumonectomy is safe and effective for non-small cell lung cancer following induction therapy. J Thorac Dis 2017;9(11):4447–53.

10. Billmeier Sarah E, Ayanian John Z, He Y, et al. Predictors of nursing home admission, severe functional impairment, or death one year after surgery for non-small cell lung cancer. Ann Surg 2013; 257(3):555–63.

11. Cykert S, Kissling G, Hansen CJ. Patient preferences regarding possible outcomes of lung resection: what outcomes should preoperative evaluations target? Chest 2000;117(6):1551–9.

12. Orringer MB, Forastiere AA, Perez-Tamayo C, et al. Chemotherapy and radiation therapy before transhiatal esophagectomy for esophageal carcinoma. Ann Thorac Surg 1990;49(3):348–54 [discussion: 354–5].

13. Sugarbaker DJ, Herndon J, Kohman LJ, et al. Results of cancer and leukemia group B protocol 8935. A multiinstitutional phase II trimodality trial for stage IIIA (N2) non-small-cell lung cancer. Cancer and Leukemia Group B Thoracic Surgery Group. J Thorac Cardiovasc Surg 1995;109(3):473–83 [discussion: 483–5].

14. Albain KS, Swann RS, Rusch VW, et al. Radiotherapy plus chemotherapy with or without surgical resection for stage III non-small cell lung cancer. Lancet 2009;374(9687):379–86.

15. Fried LP, Tangen CM, Walston J, et al. Frailty in older adults: evidence for a phenotype. J Gerontol A Biol Sci Med Sci 2001;56(3):M146–56.

16. Smart R, Carter B, McGovern J, et al. Frailty exists in younger adults admitted as surgical emergency leading to adverse outcomes. J Frailty Aging 2017; 6(4):219–23.

17. Johansen Kirsten L, Chertow Glenn M, Jin C, et al. Significance of frailty among dialysis patients. JASN 2007;18(11):2960–7.

18. Eto K, Mitsuyoshi U, Makoto K, et al. Standardization of surgical procedures to reduce risk of anastomotic leakage, reoperation, and surgical site infection in colorectal cancer surgery: a retrospective cohort study of 1189 patients. Int J Colorectal Dis 2018; 33(6):755–62.

19. Hui-Shan L, Watts JN, Peel NM, et al. Frailty and post-operative outcomes in older surgical patients: a systematic review. BMC Geriatr 2016;16(1):157.

20. Fontana L, Kennedy Brian K, Longo Valter D, et al. Medical research: treat ageing. Nature 2014; 511(7510):405–7.

21. Theou O, Rockwood Michael RH, Arnold M, et al. Disability and co-morbidity in relation to frailty: how much do they overlap? Arch Gerontol Geriatr 2012; 55(2):e1–8.

22. Hofhuis José GM, van Stel Henk F, Schrijvers Augustinus JP, et al. Changes of health-related quality of life in critically ill octogenarians: a follow-up study. Chest 2011;140(6):1473–83.

23. Bandeen-Roche K, Seplaki Christopher L, Huang J, et al. Frailty in older adults: a nationally representative profile in the United States. J Gerontol A Biol Sci Med Sci 2015;70(11):1427–34.

24. Beckert Angela K, Huisingh-Scheetz M, Thompson K, et al. Screening for frailty in thoracic surgical patients. Ann Thorac Surg 2017;103(3):956–61.

25. Won E. Issues in the management of esophageal cancer and geriatric patients. Chin Clin Oncol 2017;6(5):8.

26. Elliott Jessie A, Doyle Suzanne L, Murphy Conor F, et al. Sarcopenia: prevalence, and impact on operative and oncologic outcomes in the multimodal management of locally advanced esophageal cancer. Ann Surg 2017;266(5):822–30.

27. Rockwood K, Song X, Chris M, et al. A global clinical measure of fitness and frailty in elderly people. CMAJ 2005;173(5):489–95.

28. Rowe R, Iqbal J, Murali-krishnan R, et al. Role of frailty assessment in patients undergoing cardiac interventions. Open Heart 2014;1(1). https://doi.org/10.1136/openhrt-2013-000033.

29. McAdams-DeMarco MA, King Elizabeth A, Luo X, et al. Frailty, length of stay, and mortality in kidney transplant recipients: a national registry and prospective cohort study. Ann Surg 2017;266(6):1084–90.

30. Sheppard Vanessa B, Leigh Anne F, George L, et al. Frailty and adherence to adjuvant hormonal therapy in older women with breast cancer: CALGB protocol 369901. J Clin Oncol 2014;32(22):2318–27.

31. Searle Samuel D, Arnold M, Gahbauer Evelyne A, et al. A standard procedure for creating a frailty index. BMC Geriatr 2008;8(1):24.

32. Martin R, Karl-Günter G, Christian SC. Significance of frailty for predicting adverse clinical outcomes in different patient groups with specific medical conditions. Z Gerontol Geriatr 2016. https://doi.org/10.1007/s00391-016-1128-8.

33. Theou O, Yu Solomon CY, Rockwood K, et al. Focus on frailty: essential as the population ages. Medicine Today 2015;16(8):28–33.

34. Kaplan Stephen J, Trottman Paul A, Porteous Grete H, et al. Functional recovery after lung resection: a before and after prospective cohort study of activity. Ann Thorac Surg 2019;107(1):209–16.

35. Mohanty S, Rosenthal Ronnie A, Russell Marcia M, et al. Optimal perioperative management of the geriatric patient: a best practices guideline from the American College of Surgeons NSQIP and the American Geriatrics Society. J Am Coll Surgeons 2016;222(5):930–47.

36. Alvarez-Nebreda ML, Bentov N, Urman Richard D, et al. Recommendations for preoperative management of frailty from the society for perioperative assessment and quality improvement (SPAQI). J Clin Anesth 2018;47:33–42.

37. Arias F, Margaret W, Urman Richard D, et al. Rapid in-person cognitive screening in the preoperative setting: test considerations and recommendations from the Society for Perioperative Assessment and Quality Improvement (SPAQI). J Clin Anesth 2020;62:109724.

38. Waite I, Deshpande R, Baghai M, et al. Home-based preoperative rehabilitation (prehab) to improve physical function and reduce hospital length of stay for frail patients undergoing coronary artery bypass graft and valve surgery. J Cardiothorac Surg 2017;12(1):91.

39. Howard R, Yin Yue S, McCandless L, et al. Taking control of your surgery: impact of a prehabilitation program on major abdominal surgery. J Am Coll Surg 2019;228(1):72–80.

40. Hulzebos Erik HJ, Helders Paul JM, Favié Nine J, et al. Preoperative intensive inspiratory muscle training to prevent postoperative pulmonary complications in high-risk patients undergoing CABG surgery: a randomized clinical trial. JAMA 2006;296(15):1851–7.

41. Schmidt M, Rahel E, Kathrin S, et al. Patient empowerment improved perioperative quality of care in cancer patients aged $\geq$ 65 years - a randomized controlled trial. PLoS One 2015;10(9):e0137824.

42. Marc L, Karenovics W, Diaper J, et al. Short-term preoperative high-intensity interval training in patients awaiting lung cancer surgery: a randomized controlled trial. J Thorac Oncol 2017;12(2):323–33.

43. Hoogeboom Thomas J, Dronkers Jaap J, Hulzebos Erik HJ, et al. Merits of exercise therapy before and after major surgery. Curr Opin Anaesthesiol 2014;27(2):161–6.

44. Fairuz B, Tristan B, Debeaumont D, et al. Impact of prehabilitation on morbidity and mortality after pulmonary lobectomy by minimally invasive surgery: a cohort study. J Thorac Dis 2018;10(4):2240–8.

45. Esra P, Turna A, Gurses A, et al. The effects of preoperative short-term intense physical therapy in lung cancer patients: a randomized controlled trial. Ann Thorac Cardiovasc Surg 2011;17(5):461–8.

46. Morano Maria T, Araújo Amanda S, Nascimento Francisco B, et al. Preoperative pulmonary rehabilitation versus chest physical therapy in patients undergoing lung cancer resection: a pilot randomized controlled trial. Arch Phys Med Rehabil 2013;94(1):53–8.

47. Francesco S, Ilernando M, Raffaele C, et al. High-intensity training and cardiopulmonary exercise testing in patients with chronic obstructive pulmonary disease and non-small-cell lung cancer undergoing lobectomy. Eur J Cardiothorac Surg 2013;44(4):e260–5.

48. Roberto B, Dennis W, Novotny P, et al. Preoperative pulmonary rehabilitation before lung cancer resection: results from two randomized studies. Lung Cancer 2011;74(3):441–5.

49. Liu Z, Qiu T, Pei L, et al. Two-week multimodal prehabilitation program improves perioperative functional capability in patients undergoing thoracoscopic lobectomy for lung cancer: a randomized controlled trial. Anesth Analg 2019. https://doi.org/10.1213/ANE.0000000000004342.

50. Rosero Ilem D, Ramírez-Vélez R, Lucia A, et al. Systematic review and meta-analysis of randomized, controlled trials on preoperative physical exercise interventions in patients with non-small-cell lung cancer. Cancers (Basel) 2019;11(7). https://doi.org/10.3390/cancers11070944.

51. Nici L, Donner C, Wouters E, et al. American Thoracic Society/European Respiratory Society statement on pulmonary rehabilitation. Am J Respir Crit Care Med 2006;173(12):1390–413.

52. Ries Andrew L, Bauldoff Gerene S, Carlin Brian W, et al. Pulmonary rehabilitation: joint ACCP/AACVPR evidence-based clinical practice guidelines. Chest 2007;131(5 Suppl):4S–42S.

53. Vogelmeier Claus F, Criner Gerard J, Martinez Fernando J, et al. Global strategy for the diagnosis, management, and prevention of chronic obstructive lung disease 2017 report. GOLD executive summary. Am J Respir Crit Care Med 2017;195(5):557–82.

54. Kaymaz D. Comprehensive multidisciplinary pulmonary rehabilitation is an effective treatment strategy in old elderly patients with COPD. Acta Med 2017;(2):321–7.

55. Lin D, Ma L, Ye T, et al. Results of neoadjuvant therapy followed by esophagectomy for patients with locally advanced thoracic esophageal squamous cell carcinoma. J Thorac Dis 2017;9(2):318–26.

56. van Hagen P, Hulshof MCCM, van Lanschot JJB, et al. Preoperative chemoradiotherapy for esophageal or junctional cancer. N Engl J Med 2012;366(22):2074–84.

57. Minnella Enrico M, Rashami A, Sarah-Eve L, et al. Effect of exercise and nutrition prehabilitation on functional capacity in esophagogastric cancer surgery: a randomized clinical trial. JAMA Surg 2018;153(12):1081–9.

58. Soares SM, Nucci LB, da Silva MM, et al. Pulmonary function and physical performance outcomes with preoperative physical therapy in upper abdominal surgery: a randomized controlled trial. Clin Rehabil 2013. https://doi.org/10.1177/0269215512471063.

59. Prehabilitation for esophagectomy - Doganay - Journal of Thoracic Disease. Available at: http://jtd.amegroups.com/article/view/27647/20650. Accessed March 27, 2020.

60. PREhabilitation for improving QUality of recovery after ELective cardiac surgery (PREQUEL) study: protocol of a randomised controlled trial. - PubMed - NCBI. Available at: https://www.ncbi.nlm.nih.gov/pubmed/31092666. Accessed March 27, 2020.

61. Lai Y, Huang J, Yang M, et al. Seven-day intensive preoperative rehabilitation for elderly patients with lung cancer: a randomized controlled trial. J Surg Res 2017;209:30–6.

62. Navarro-Ripoll R, Arguis MJ, Coca-Martínez M, et al. Multimodal prehabilitation to improve functional capacity in cardiac surgery: feasibility and safety. J Cardiothorac Vasc Anesth 2018;32:S77–8.

63. McIsaac Daniel I, Saunders C, Hladkowicz E, et al. PREHAB study: a protocol for a prospective randomised clinical trial of exercise therapy for people living with frailty having cancer surgery. BMJ Open 2018;8(6):e022057.

64. Bravo-Iñiguez C, Perez MM, Armstrong Katherine W, et al. Surgical resection of lung cancer in the elderly. Thorac Surg Clin 2014;24(4):371–81.

65. Fleisher LA, Fleischmann KE, Auerbach AD, et al. 2014 ACC/AHA guideline on perioperative cardiovascular evaluation and management of patients undergoing noncardiac surgery. J Am Coll Cardiol 2014;64(22):e77–137. Available at: http://www.onlinejacc.org/content/64/22/e77. Accessed March 27, 2020.

Enhanced Recovery After Thoracic Surgery

Nathan Haywood, MD[a], Ian Nickel, MD[a], Aimee Zhang, MD[a], Matthew Byler, MD, MBA[a], Erik Scott, MD[a], Walker Julliard, MD[a], Randal S. Blank, MD, PhD[b], Linda W. Martin, MD, MPH[a,c],*

KEYWORDS

- Thoracic surgery • Prehabilitation • Opioid sparing • Early ambulation • Early enteral nutrition

KEY POINTS

- Enhanced recovery pathways (ERPs), used across multiple surgical subspecialties, are multidisciplinary approaches to the delivery of perioperative care that are designed to return patients to baseline as quickly as possible.
- Although small variations exist between programs, core tenets of thoracic surgery ERP have been implemented in several centers over the last few years.
- Evidence of the benefit of thoracic ERP has started to emerge in terms of clinical outcomes and health care–associated cost.

INTRODUCTION

To lessen the physiologic and psychological stress of patients undergoing surgery, protocolized approaches using multidisciplinary delivery of care have been adopted. Coined enhanced recovery after surgery (ERAS), the goal includes returning patients to their preoperative baselines as early as possible. Enhanced recovery pathways (ERPs) were initially described in colorectal surgery more than 20 years ago and have since been implemented across multiple surgical subspecialties.[1] Protocols encompass the preoperative, intraoperative, and postoperative periods and have shown benefit in patient outcomes as well as health care–associated cost.[1] Although variations exist between institutions, consistent core tenets include preoperative patient education, avoidance of prolonged preoperative fasting, limiting intravenous fluid administration, multimodal opioid-sparing analgesia, and early ambulation.[2]

Surgical access for thoracic surgery requires one of the most painful incisions even when a minimally invasive approach is used.[3] In addition, lung surgery is associated with significant risks of postoperative morbidity.[4] As such, patients undergoing thoracic surgery encounter numerous psychological and physiologic stressors. In the past several years, ERPs have been developed in thoracic surgery (**Box 1**). Although similar in some aspects to earlier described fast-track thoracic surgery pathways, thoracic ERP places heavier focus on the quality rather than the speed of recovery, achievement of homeostasis, multidisciplinary delivery of care, preoperative education, and opioid-sparing pain management.[3] Evidence of the benefit of thoracic ERP has started to emerge.[5] However, implementation of such a program may seem daunting. This article presents common components of an ERP for thoracic surgery and discusses contemporary outcomes. Although ERPs for

[a] Division of Thoracic & Cardiovascular Surgery, Department of Surgery, University of Virginia Health System, 1215 Lee Street, Charlottesville, VA 22908-0679, USA; [b] Division of General Anesthesiology, Department of Anesthesiology, University of Virginia Health System, 1215 Lee Street, Charlottesville, VA 22908-0679, USA; [c] Thoracic Surgery, University of Virginia Health System, 1215 Lee Street, Charlottesville, VA 22908-0679, USA
* Corresponding author. Thoracic Surgery, University of Virginia Health System, 1215 Lee Street, Charlottesville, VA 22908-0679.
E-mail address: LM6YB@virginia.edu

Thorac Surg Clin 30 (2020) 259–267
https://doi.org/10.1016/j.thorsurg.2020.04.005
1547-4127/20/© 2020 Elsevier Inc. All rights reserved.

Box 1
ERAS Society and European Society of Thoracic Surgeons guidelines for enhanced recovery after lung surgery

Preoperative phase

  Preadmission information, education, counseling

  Preoperative nutrition screening and counseling

  Smoking cessation

  Alcohol dependency management

  Anemia identified, investigated, corrected

  Prehabilitation, pulmonary rehabilitation

Perioperative phase

  Clear fluids until 2 hours before; oral carbohydrate load

  Venous thromboembolism prophylaxis

  Antibiotic prophylaxis and skin preparation

  Prevent intraoperative hypothermia

  Anesthesia: lung-protective strategies; use regional and general anesthesia together

  Postoperative nausea and vomiting control

  Regional anesthesia and pain relief: multimodal opioid sparing

  Fluid management: discontinue intravenous fluids as soon as possible and replace with oral fluids

  Atrial fibrillation prevention strategy should be in place

  Surgical technique: muscle sparing if thoracotomy needed, video-assisted thoracoscopic surgery for early stage when possible

Postoperative phase

  Chest tubes: avoid external suction, remove as soon as possible, use single tube

  Urinary drainage: avoid if possible, reasonable to use if epidural, spinal

  Early mobilization and physical therapy within 24 hours

Adapted from Batchelor TJP, Rasburn NJ, Abdelnour-Berchtold E, et al. Guidelines for enhanced recovery after lung surgery: recommendations of the Enhanced Recovery After Surgery (ERAS®) Society and the European Society of Thoracic Surgeons (ESTS). Eur J Cardiothorac Surg. 2019;55(1):93–4; with permission.

esophageal surgery have also emerged, the focus here is on lung surgery. Common trends are discussed, as well as our institutional experience.

PREOPERATIVE PHASE
Preadmission Education and Information

ERPs place heavy emphasis on the intraoperative and postoperative care of thoracic surgical patients. However, preoperative optimization and preparation are equally important for truly enhanced recovery (ER). The provision of tailored information to the patients about the procedure and recovery process has proved to be fundamental to the optimization process.[6] Delivery should be multimodal with a combination of personal counseling, printed materials, and/or electronic resources designed to enhance patient understanding. It is our practice to provide patients with a preassembled folder during a preoperative clinic visit. This material serves to achieve the following goals: (1) to prepare and manage patient expectations for the preoperative, intraoperative, and postoperative phases; (2) to encourage active participation of the patients in their care; and (3) to alleviate patient anxiety about the accelerated pace of recovery and the unknown.

Smoking Cessation

Smoking has obvious long-term risks and also represents a considerable source of short-term risk for postoperative complications in thoracic surgery.[7] The provision of resources for smoking cessation is essential for patients who need thoracic surgery. The current recommendations suggest intervention initiated at least 4 to 8 weeks before surgery, but, in general, smoking cessation should be recommended regardless of timing.[8]

Exercise Capacity and Prehabilitation

Preoperative optimization of functional status and physical reserve has been advocated to better allow patients to withstand the stress of the perioperative period and return to normal activity (**Fig. 1**).[9] Coined prehabilitation, the goal is to increase preoperative functional level with exercise training and nutritional supplementation.[9] Thoracic ERPs have adapted prehabilitation because poor preoperative exercise capacity in patients undergoing lung surgery has been associated with increased postoperative complications and increased length of stay (LOS).[1] Although many programs incorporate some form of exercise prehabilitation, outcome improvements following lung cancer surgery have yet to be established. During the preoperative visit at our institution, patients are given information about preoperative exercise and are encouraged to be as active as possible leading up to surgery.

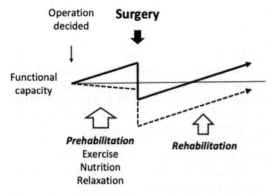

Fig. 1. Theoretic model showing the benefit of prehabilitation on functional capacity before and after surgery. (*From* Kawaguchi M, Ida M, Naito Y. The role of Perioperative Surgical Home on health and longevity in society: importance of the surgical prehabilitation program. J Anesth. 2017;31(3):319–24; with permission.)

Nutrition and Carbohydrate Loading

Essential principles of the preoperative ERP include nutritional optimization and avoidance of long-term fasting.[10] European Society for Clinical Nutrition and Metabolism guidelines recommend screening patients preoperatively in an effort to identify malnutrition (weight loss >10%–15% within 6 months; body mass index <18.5; serum albumin level <3 g/dL) and, if indicated, provide nutritional support for 10 to 14 days before major surgery.[10] Fasting beginning at midnight before the operation is no longer recommended and can lead to dehydration and insulin resistance, which is exacerbated by the metabolic stress associated with surgery.[11–13] Compared with a traditional fasting period, a Cochrane Review in the early 2000s showed no increased aspiration risk with oral fluids 2 to 3 hours before surgery.[12,13] Preoperative oral carbohydrate loading 2 hours before surgery, initially in the laparoscopic cholecystectomy population, was found to mitigate postoperative nausea, vomiting, and pain, and to decrease overall LOS.[11,12] Pachella and colleagues[14] (2019) showed that carbohydrate loading 2 hours before thoracic surgery decreased use of opioids and antiemetic medications in the immediate postoperative period. There are numerous ERAS drinks available but no specific ones have been shown to improve outcomes. Our institution uses regular 591-mL (20-oz) Gatorade because of low cost and availability.

INTRAOPERATIVE PHASE
Preemptive Analgesia and Regional Nerve Blockade

The authors routinely give oral acetaminophen, gabapentin, and celecoxib on arrival to surgical preparation area. We do not use celecoxib with renal insufficiency or planned pleurodesis. Regional nerve blockade is preferred to the use of opioids for preemptive pain control.[15] Thoracic epidural analgesia has been used for thoracotomy in thoracic ERPs[1,16,17]; however, it is associated with increased rate of postoperative hypotension, urinary retention, and weakness. Such complications are not congruent with the early mobilization goal of ERP.[1,17] Alternative strategies with fewer side effects include paravertebral and intercostal nerve blockade.[18,19] Elastomeric catheters containing local anesthetics are expensive, prone to occlusion, and have conflicting reports regarding efficacy in controlling postthoracotomy pain.[15,18,20] Liposomal bupivacaine (Exparel, Pacira Pharmaceuticals, Parsippany, NJ) has been used for regional nerve blockade in thoracic surgery.[15,21] This formula provides up to 96 hours of bupivacaine release from liposomal vesicles, obviating continuous infusion catheters.[15] Following lung resection, Rice and colleagues[15] (2015) showed similar pain scores and decreased LOS in patients undergoing intercostal nerve blockade with liposomal bupivacaine compared with thoracic epidural anesthesia. Similar findings have been previously reported.[19] At our institution, preemptive regional nerve blockade includes posterior intercostal nerve blockade of interspaces 3 to 10 using dilute liposomal bupivacaine injected transcutaneously, at the start of the operation.[22] We have found the best results when done with video-assisted thoracoscopic surgery (VATS) guidance, regardless of plans for VATS or open surgery. Postoperative analgesia is further augmented with the intrathecal administration of preservative-free morphine for patients requiring thoracotomy incisions and anatomic lung resections.

Deep Vein Thrombosis Prophylaxis, Skin Preparation, and Antibiotic Prophylaxis

All patients in thoracic ERP should have mechanical deep vein thrombosis (DVT) prophylaxis with sequential compression devices or foot pumps.[16] Pharmacologic DVT prophylaxis (low-molecular-weight heparin or unfractionated heparin) should be administered in patients not at high risk of bleeding.[16] Preoperative intravenous antibiotic prophylaxis, usually a cephalosporin, should be administered no more than 60 minutes before incision and redosed appropriately intraoperatively.[16] Extended antibiotic prophylaxis following surgery has not been shown to improve outcomes.[16] Hair removal should be as limited as possible.[16] Chlorhexidine-alcohol solutions are preferred, because they have been shown to decrease surgical site infection compared with povidone-iodine solutions.[16,23]

Intraoperative Anesthesia

Short-acting anesthetic agents permitting early extubation are a mainstay of thoracic ERPs.[1,16,17,24] Compared with intravenous anesthesia, volatile inhaled anesthetic agents such as sevoflurane and desflurane have been shown to suppress the local alveolar inflammatory response associated with one-lung ventilation.[25] However, total intravenous anesthesia with propofol has been associated with lower rates of postoperative nausea and vomiting.[26] As such, acceptable anesthetic includes short-acting volatile or intravenous anesthetics used individually or in combination.[16]

Intraoperative multimodal analgesia with minimal use of opiates is a core component of ERPs. Intraoperative ketamine is used as part of our thoracic ERP program.[3] Although its specific benefit in thoracic surgery has not yet been clearly elucidated, ketamine combined with regional anesthesia has been shown to control perioperative pain in major digestive surgery.[27] The strategy at our institution includes induction with appropriate anesthetic and adjunctive agents followed by maintenance anesthesia with sevoflurane and ketamine.[3] Opiate use is minimized and only administered with approval by an attending physician.[3]

Intraoperative Fluid Management

Perioperative fluid management in thoracic surgery is of critical importance because liberal use can increase risk of pulmonary complications such as acute respiratory distress syndrome. There is also concern that excessive volume restricting can lead to hypovolemic complications such as acute kidney injury.[1,16,17,24] In a retrospective analysis of 1442 patients undergoing thoracic surgery, Ahn and colleagues[28] (2016) showed that fluid-restrictive approaches (<3 mL/kg/h) were not associated with increased development of acute kidney injury. At present, most thoracic ER programs use intraoperative balanced crystalloid in a restrictive manor (<3 mL/kg/h, <2 L total intraoperatively).[3,24]

Intraoperative Ventilation

Perhaps in no other population is it more important to limit ventilator-associated pulmonary complications than in those undergoing thoracic surgery. For this reason, a focus of thoracic ER programs is a lung-protective ventilation strategy.[1,16,17,24] Because one-lung ventilation is typically required for optimal surgical exposure in lung surgery, lung-protective strategies have focused on limiting tidal volumes and airway driving pressure in the ventilated lung and preventing hypoxia and other complications associated with collapse in the nonventilated lung.[16,24] Current strategies include limiting tidal volume to 4 to 5 mL/kg predicted body weight in the ventilated lung with positive end-expiratory pressure to limit hypoxia.[16,24] In addition, low-level continuous positive airway pressure to the collapsed lung has been shown to decrease inflammatory response associated with complete collapse.[29]

POSTOPERATIVE PHASE
Postoperative Analgesia

Effective postoperative pain management is a prerequisite for adequate pulmonary mechanical function and hygiene, and preventing postoperative atelectasis, pneumonia, and other complications. The authors use a ketamine infusion (0.1–0.5 mg/kg) for 24 to 48 hours following surgery.[30] At this dose, ketamine augments postoperative pain control without causing adverse hemodynamic effects or respiratory depression.[31] Occasionally patients experience mild hallucinations or diplopia, which is usually well tolerated and resolves with discontinuation of the infusion. With the use of these adjuncts as well as scheduled oral analgesics (acetaminophen, gabapentin, and nonsteroidal antiinflammatory drugs), opioids can be reserved to treat breakthrough pain.[1,3]

Bladder Drainage

Urinary catheter removal on the first postoperative day should occur even in the presence of a thoracic epidural or spinal morphine to avoid infection and to optimize patient comfort.[32] This technique is often used with bladder scan urinary retention protocols and, in our program, the routine administration of tamsulosin for all male patients older than 50 years.[3,33] The successful implementation of early, protocol-driven removal of indwelling urinary catheters as part of ERPs decreases LOS.[30,33]

Postoperative Diet

ERPs across specialties share the goal of maintaining homeostasis to avoid catabolism, protein loss, and cellular dysfunction.[34] Early discontinuation of intravenous fluids and initiation of oral feeding after surgery are important elements of this strategy. Thoracic ERPs permit diet advancement as tolerated within an hour or two of surgery. ERPs typically include a multimodal approach to prevent postoperative nausea and vomiting by both nonpharmacologic (preoperative carbohydrate loading, avoidance of crystalloid overload) and pharmacologic (avoidance of opiates, regular administration of antiemetics, intraoperative dexamethasone 4 mg) measures, as well as aggressive inpatient and discharge oral bowel regimens.[3,35]

Chest Tube Management

Chest tubes are a necessary evil of thoracic surgery because they impair mobilization and increase LOS and cost.[1,36] The application of external suction may also exacerbate air leak duration[37] and further limit mobilization by anchoring the patient to the suction source.[5] Removal of chest tubes objectively improves ventilatory function, as measured by expiratory volume and vital capacity, and reduces chest pain after forced thoracic surgery.[38] Historically, chest tube management was based on surgeon experience and preference, with most surgeons preferring to leave the chest tube in place until the volume of drainage decreased below an arbitrary threshold (often 250 mL/d or less).[39] More aggressive chest tube removal strategies have shown similar outcomes with fluid thresholds of 450 to 500 mL/d following VATS and thoracotomy.[40,41] For our institutional ERP, chest tubes are placed on water seal within 12 hours, unless there is a major air leak. Chest tubes are removed when there is no air leak, bloody output, or chyle. The total volume of chest tube output and postoperative days since surgery are not factors in the decision.[3]

Postoperative Atrial Fibrillation

Postoperative atrial fibrillation (POAF) is the most common arrhythmia after thoracic surgery.[42] It has been associated with increased mortality, increased hospital and intensive care unit LOS, and higher resource use.[36,42,43] American Association for Thoracic Surgery (AATS) guidelines on the prevention of POAF include a class I recommendation for continuing the patient's home β-adrenergic antagonists and a class IIb recommendation for repleting low serum magnesium levels. In addition, intravenous amiodarone or diltiazem administration for POAF prophylaxis is given a class IIa recommendation.[44] Three meta-analyses have been performed on the topic of medical prophylaxis for POAF after general thoracic surgery, all of which show that calcium channel blockers (CCBs; eg, diltiazem), amiodarone, β-blockers, and magnesium replacement are all effective agents for prevention of POAF.[45–47]

In 2017, Zhao and colleagues[45] performed a meta-analysis that evaluated 22 studies that compared pharmacoprophylaxis for prevention of POAF. In addition to confirming the aforementioned recommendations, they also showed that prophylaxis with β-adrenergic antagonists was well tolerated and may be more effective than CCBs or amiodarone. β-Adrenergic antagonists were not included in the 2014 AATS guidelines for prevention of POAF; however, in 2016, a prospective randomized controlled trial by Cardinale and colleagues[48] showed metoprolol to be effective in reducing incidence of POAF. Our practice is to resume home β-adrenergic antagonist therapy. Other patients are stratified to either high-risk or low-risk groups, with high-risk (defined as age >50 years having either thoracotomy or anatomic resection) patients receiving postoperative diltiazem for prevention of POAF.

OUTCOMES
Patient Outcomes

Although a predecessor of contemporary thoracic ERP, fast-tracking for pulmonary resection was described by Cerfolio and colleagues[49] as early as 2001. An assessment of patient outcomes following a fast-track clinical pathway for lung resection was described in 2008.[50] In a prospective randomized trial, Muehling and colleagues[50] reported decreased pulmonary complications associated with a fast-track pathway for lung resection. Overall morbidity and mortality were unchanged.[50] Madani and colleagues[33] (2015) later showed a decreased postoperative complication rate without change in early mortality in an ERP for open lobectomy. Similar findings were shown by Paci and colleagues[51] (2017) for elective lung resection, including both VATS and thoracotomy. When VATS lobectomy was evaluated independently, Brunelli and colleagues[52] (2017) showed no difference in postoperative complications or early mortality associated with implementation of an ERP. Most of these pathways used conservative chest tube management, epidural pain control, and patient-controlled anesthesia,[50] emphasizing that the components of published ERPs vary widely and, not surprisingly, the impact on outcomes varies as well.[3,21] In one of the largest published studies on ERP in lung cancer resection, Van Haren and colleagues[4] (2018) showed improved cardiac and pulmonary complication rates following thoracotomy.[4] However, a similar benefit was not shown in the minimally invasive cohort. Evidence is emerging that thoracic ERPs decrease complication rate following thoracotomy, but a similar benefit in VATS has not been consistently shown, perhaps because there is less room for improvement. The authors recently published a comparison of VATS and open lobectomies on an ERP, which suggests the ERP negates differences between VATS and open lobectomy for traditional surgical outcomes, including rate of postoperative complications. Because more total nodes and nodal stations were assessed with thoracotomy, this factor may have important oncologic implications.[53] Rogers and colleagues[35] (2018) showed a positive association between compliance with major ERP core tenets and decreased morbidity following lung cancer resection. It is unclear at this time whether the benefit stems from specific components of thoracic ERP or all changes in aggregate.[5] Detailed study of patient outcomes related to ERP components and compliance will be critical for improvement as these programs continue to evolve.

Patient-Reported Outcomes and Length of Stay

Patient-reported outcomes (PROs) are measures of patient physical and psychosocial well-being that are directly reported by patients.[54] These metrics are increasingly used for quality of care.[54,55] A recent review of thoracic ERP by Medbery and colleagues[54] (2019) highlights the critical need to include PROs alongside traditionally reported measures of morbidity and mortality.

An important determinant in patient satisfaction is LOS. Grigor and colleagues[55] (2017) showed that prolonged LOS following lung cancer surgery was associated with a marked decreased in patient experience. Following implementation of a thoracic ERP protocol following thoracotomy, several centers have shown a decrease in postoperative LOS without increasing the readmission rate.[3,4,30,33,35] Madani and colleagues[33] (2015) showed a decrease in median LOS from 7 to 6 days in open lobectomy following ER protocol implementation. Other centers have since shown even greater benefit by focusing on early chest tube removal and avoidance of epidural use.[35] For example, 1-year analysis at our institution revealed a decrease in median LOS from 6 to 4 days following implementation of ERP for thoracotomy.[3] Similar findings have not yet been shown for all ERPs following VATS, perhaps because LOS is already short in this cohort, but some investigators have shown improvements even in a VATS cohort.[3,52,56,57] Decreased LOS not only leads to patient satisfaction but also translates into decreased resource use and health care–associated costs.

Return to Intended Oncologic Therapy

Cancer surgery is frequently just 1 part of multidisciplinary oncologic care. Full recovery after surgery is a key factor in receiving all prescribed cancer treatment and has been shown to improve disease-free and overall survival.[58] Standard of care in the treatment of stage II and higher non–small cell lung cancer includes adjuvant chemotherapy.[59] Achievement of good performance status (Eastern Cooperative Oncology Group 0) is generally required before initiation of chemotherapy. The decrease in postoperative morbidity, lower pain scores, and quicker return to baseline associated with thoracic ERPs positively affects the ability of patients to initiate and complete this critical component of care.[59] Nelson and colleagues[59] (2019) showed shortened time to adjuvant chemotherapy and higher rate of completing 4 or more chemotherapy cycles following adoption of a thoracic ERP. Impact on survival has not yet been reported in a lung cancer population.

Cost

Like other surgical disciplines, the adoption of thoracic ERP seems to be associated with a durable decrease in overall health system cost. The development of ERPs across multiple surgical disciplines and service lines has led to a decrease in hospital cost.[34,51] ERPs within thoracic surgery are no exception.[51,60,61] Although predating the current ERP era, standardized clinical care pathways reduced hospital costs following anatomic lung resections as early as 1997.[60–62] A Johns Hopkins University study reported hospital savings of approximately $4000 with the implementation of a standardized pathway following major pulmonary anatomic resection.[61,63] Similarly, decreased costs were shown using standardized pathways following VATS pulmonary resection the early 2000s.[60,63] Following the implementation of thoracic ERP protocol and ERPs, both VATS and thoracotomy remain associated with lower hospital costs. Mean inflation-adjusted hospital costs significantly decreased by about $5500 for VATS and almost $16,000 for major thoracotomy 1 year after the implementation of thoracic ERP at our institution.[3] Another study, by Paci and colleagues[51] (2017), showed no change in total institutional or health system costs following implementation of thoracic ERP, but it did show a reduction in societal cost by almost $4500 (Canadian). This finding is likely caused by quicker return to baseline and less productivity loss after discharge. In addition, although total institutional costs were unchanged, intensive care unit and ward costs were significantly lower following implementation, in part because of shorter hospital LOS.[51]

SUMMARY

Numerous studies have shown the clinical and economic benefits of ERPs for lung surgery. Areas of interest and ongoing study in thoracic ERP include the potential effect of opioid-sparing analgesia on chronic postthoracotomy pain, new opioid dependence, cancer recurrence, and the effect of ERP on PROs and quality-of-life measures. Continued multidisciplinary review and protocol revision are of paramount importance for ERP improvement. It is likely that the full potential of thoracic ERPs has not yet been realized and that more widespread adoption and study of these pathways will lead to further improvements in care and outcomes.

DISCLOSURE

The authors have nothing to disclose.

REFERENCES

1. Dinic VD, Stojanovic MD, Markovic D, et al. Enhanced recovery in thoracic surgery: a review. Front Med (Lausanne) 2018;5:14.
2. Thiele RH, Raghunathan K, Brudney CS, et al. American Society for Enhanced Recovery (ASER) and Perioperative Quality Initiative (POQI) joint consensus statement on perioperative fluid management within an enhanced recovery pathway for colorectal surgery. Perioper Med (Lond) 2016; 5:24.
3. Martin LW, Sarosiek BM, Harrison MA, et al. Implementing a thoracic enhanced recovery program: lessons learned in the first year. Ann Thorac Surg 2018;105(6):1597–604.
4. Van Haren RM, Mehran RJ, Mena GE, et al. Enhanced recovery decreases pulmonary and cardiac complications after thoracotomy for lung cancer. Ann Thorac Surg 2018;106(1):272–9.
5. Batchelor TJP, Ljungqvist O. A surgical perspective of ERAS guidelines in thoracic surgery. Curr Opin Anaesthesiol 2019;32(1):17–22.
6. Jankowski CJ. Preparing the patient for enhanced recovery after surgery. Int Anesthesiology Clin 2017;55(4):12–20.
7. Turan A, Mascha EJ, Roberman D, et al. Smoking and perioperative outcomes. Anesthesiology 2011; 114(4):837–46.
8. Thomsen T, Villebro N, Moller AM. Interventions for preoperative smoking cessation. Cochrane Database Syst Rev 2014;(3):CD002294.
9. Kawaguchi M, Ida M, Naito Y. The role of Perioperative Surgical Home on health and longevity in society: importance of the surgical prehabilitation program. J Anesth 2017;31(3):319–24.
10. Weimann A, Braga M, Harsanyi L, et al. ESPEN guidelines on enteral nutrition: surgery including organ transplantation. Clin Nutr 2006;25(2): 224–44.
11. Singh BN, Dahiya D, Bagaria D, et al. Effects of preoperative carbohydrates drinks on immediate postoperative outcome after day care laparoscopic cholecystectomy. Surg Endosc 2015;29(11):3267–72.
12. Kratzing C. Pre-operative nutrition and carbohydrate loading. Proc Nutr Soc 2011;70(3):311–5.
13. Brady M, Kinn S, Stuart P. Preoperative fasting for adults to prevent perioperative complications. Cochrane Database Syst Rev 2003;(4):CD004423.
14. Pachella LA, Mehran RJ, Curtin K, et al. Preoperative carbohydrate loading in patients undergoing thoracic surgery: a quality-improvement project. J Perianesth Nurs 2019;34(6):1250–6.
15. Rice DC, Cata JP, Mena GE, et al. Posterior intercostal nerve block with liposomal bupivacaine: an alternative to thoracic epidural analgesia. Ann Thorac Surg 2015;99(6):1953–60.
16. Batchelor TJP, Rasburn NJ, Abdelnour-Berchtold E, et al. Guidelines for enhanced recovery after lung surgery: recommendations of the Enhanced Recovery After Surgery (ERAS(R)) Society and the European Society of Thoracic Surgeons (ESTS). Eur J Cardiothorac Surg 2019;55(1):91–115.
17. Jones NL, Edmonds L, Ghosh S, et al. A review of enhanced recovery for thoracic anaesthesia and surgery. Anaesthesia 2013;68(2):179–89.
18. Jung J, Park SY, Haam S. Efficacy of subpleural continuous infusion of local anesthetics after thoracoscopic pulmonary resection for primary lung cancer compared to intravenous patient-controlled analgesia. J Thorac Dis 2016;8(7):1814–9.
19. Khalil KG, Boutrous ML, Irani AD, et al. Operative intercostal nerve blocks with long-acting bupivacaine liposome for pain control after thoracotomy. Ann Thorac Surg 2015;100(6):2013–8.
20. Gebhardt R, Mehran RJ, Soliz J, et al. Epidural versus ON-Q local anesthetic-infiltrating catheter for post-thoracotomy pain control. J Cardiothorac Vasc Anesth 2013;27(3):423–6.
21. Mehran RJ, Walsh GL, Zalpour A, et al. Intercostal nerve blocks with liposomal bupivacaine: demonstration of safety, and potential benefits. Semin Thorac Cardiovasc Surg 2017;29(4):531–7.
22. Martin LW, Mehran RJ. Intercostal nerve blockade for thoracic surgery with liposomal bupivacaine: the devil is in the details. J Thorac Dis 2019; 11(Suppl 9):S1202–5.
23. Darouiche RO, Wall MJ Jr, Itani KM, et al. Chlorhexidine-alcohol versus povidone-iodine for surgical-site antisepsis. N Engl J Med 2010;362(1):18–26.
24. Loop T. Fast track in thoracic surgery and anaesthesia: update of concepts. Curr Opin Anaesthesiol 2016;29(1):20–5.

25. Schilling T, Kozian A, Senturk M, et al. Effects of volatile and intravenous anesthesia on the alveolar and systemic inflammatory response in thoracic surgical patients. Anesthesiology 2011;115(1):65–74.

26. Kumar G, Stendall C, Mistry R, et al. A comparison of total intravenous anaesthesia using propofol with sevoflurane or desflurane in ambulatory surgery: systematic review and meta-analysis. Anaesthesia 2014;69(10):1138–50.

27. Lavand'homme P, De Kock M, Waterloos H. Intraoperative epidural analgesia combined with ketamine provides effective preventive analgesia in patients undergoing major digestive surgery. Anesthesiology 2005;103(4):813–20.

28. Ahn HJ, Kim JA, Lee AR, et al. The risk of acute kidney injury from fluid restriction and hydroxyethyl starch in thoracic surgery. Anesth Analg 2016; 122(1):186–93.

29. Verhage RJ, Boone J, Rijkers GT, et al. Reduced local immune response with continuous positive airway pressure during one-lung ventilation for oesophagectomy. Br J Anaesth 2014;112(5):920–8.

30. Semenkovich TR, Hudson JL, Subramanian M, et al. Enhanced Recovery After Surgery (ERAS) in thoracic surgery. Semin Thorac Cardiovasc Surg 2018;30(3):342–9.

31. Assouline B, Tramer MR, Kreienbuhl L, et al. Benefit and harm of adding ketamine to an opioid in a patient-controlled analgesia device for the control of postoperative pain: systematic review and meta-analyses of randomized controlled trials with trial sequential analyses. Pain 2016;157(12):2854–64.

32. Wald HL, Ma A, Bratzler DW, et al. Indwelling urinary catheter use in the postoperative period: analysis of the national surgical infection prevention project data. Arch Surg 2008;143(6):551–7.

33. Madani A, Fiore JF Jr, Wang Y, et al. An enhanced recovery pathway reduces duration of stay and complications after open pulmonary lobectomy. Surgery 2015;158(4):899–908 [discussion: 908–10].

34. Ljungqvist O, Scott M, Fearon KC. Enhanced recovery after surgery: a review. JAMA Surg 2017;152(3): 292–8.

35. Rogers LJ, Bleetman D, Messenger DE, et al. The impact of enhanced recovery after surgery (ERAS) protocol compliance on morbidity from resection for primary lung cancer. J Thorac Cardiovasc Surg 2018;155(4):1843–52.

36. Irshad K, Feldman LS, Chu VF, et al. Causes of increased length of hospitalization on a general thoracic surgery service: a prospective observational study. Can J Surg 2002;45(4):264–8.

37. Marshall MB, Deeb ME, Bleier JI, et al. Suction vs water seal after pulmonary resection: a randomized prospective study. Chest 2002;121(3):831–5.

38. Refai M, Brunelli A, Salati M, et al. The impact of chest tube removal on pain and pulmonary function after pulmonary resection. Eur J Cardiothorac Surg 2012;41(4):820–2 [discussion: 823].

39. Cerfolio RJ, Bryant AS. The management of chest tubes after pulmonary resection. Thorac Surg Clin 2010;20(3):399–405.

40. Bjerregaard LS, Jensen K, Petersen RH, et al. Early chest tube removal after video-assisted thoracic surgery lobectomy with serous fluid production up to 500 ml/day. Eur J Cardiothorac Surg 2014;45(2): 241–6.

41. Cerfolio RJ, Bryant AS. Results of a prospective algorithm to remove chest tubes after pulmonary resection with high output. J Thorac Cardiovasc Surg 2008;135(2):269–73.

42. Vaporciyan AA, Correa AM, Rice DC, et al. Risk factors associated with atrial fibrillation after noncardiac thoracic surgery: analysis of 2588 patients. J Thorac Cardiovasc Surg 2004;127(3):779–86.

43. Imperatori A, Mariscalco G, Riganti G, et al. Atrial fibrillation after pulmonary lobectomy for lung cancer affects long-term survival in a prospective single-center study. J Cardiothorac Surg 2012;7:4.

44. Frendl G, Sodickson AC, Chung MK, et al. 2014 AATS guidelines for the prevention and management of perioperative atrial fibrillation and flutter for thoracic surgical procedures. J Thorac Cardiovasc Surg 2014;148(3):e153–93.

45. Zhao BC, Huang TY, Deng QW, et al. Prophylaxis against atrial fibrillation after general thoracic surgery: trial sequential analysis and network meta-analysis. Chest 2017;151(1):149–59.

46. Riber LP, Larsen TB, Christensen TD. Postoperative atrial fibrillation prophylaxis after lung surgery: systematic review and meta-analysis. Ann Thorac Surg 2014;98(6):1989–97.

47. Sedrakyan A, Treasure T, Browne J, et al. Pharmacologic prophylaxis for postoperative atrial tachyarrhythmia in general thoracic surgery: evidence from randomized clinical trials. J Thorac Cardiovasc Surg 2005;129(5):997–1005.

48. Cardinale D, Sandri MT, Colombo A, et al. Prevention of atrial fibrillation in high-risk patients undergoing lung cancer surgery: the PRESAGE trial. Ann Surg 2016;264(2):244–51.

49. Cerfolio RJ, Pickens A, Bass C, et al. Fast-tracking pulmonary resections. J Thorac Cardiovasc Surg 2001;122(2):318–24.

50. Muehling BM, Halter GL, Schelzig H, et al. Reduction of postoperative pulmonary complications after lung surgery using a fast track clinical pathway. Eur J Cardiothorac Surg 2008;34(1):174–80.

51. Paci P, Madani A, Lee L, et al. Economic impact of an enhanced recovery pathway for lung resection. Ann Thorac Surg 2017;104(3):950–7.

52. Brunelli A, Thomas C, Dinesh P, et al. Enhanced recovery pathway versus standard care in patients

undergoing video-assisted thoracoscopic lobectomy. J Thorac Cardiovasc Surg 2017;154(6): 2084–90.

53. Krebs ED, Mehaffey JH, Sarosiek BM, et al. Is less really more? Reexamining video-assisted thoracoscopic versus open lobectomy in the setting of an enhanced recovery protocol. J Thorac Cardiovasc Surg 2019; 159(1):284–94.e1.

54. Medbery RL, Fernandez FG, Khullar OV. ERAS and patient reported outcomes in thoracic surgery: a review of current data. J Thorac Dis 2019;11(Suppl 7): S976–86.

55. Grigor EJM, Ivanovic J, Anstee C, et al. Impact of adverse events and length of stay on patient experience after lung cancer resection. Ann Thorac Surg 2017;104(2):382–8.

56. Khandhar SJ, Schatz CL, Collins DT, et al. Thoracic enhanced recovery with ambulation after surgery: a 6-year experience. Eur J Cardiothorac Surg 2018; 53(6):1192–8.

57. Huang H, Ma H, Chen S. Enhanced recovery after surgery using uniportal video-assisted thoracic surgery for lung cancer: A preliminary study. Thorac Cancer 2018;9(1):83–7.

58. Aloia TA, Zimmitti G, Conrad C, et al. Return to intended oncologic treatment (RIOT): a novel metric for evaluating the quality of oncosurgical therapy for malignancy. J Surg Oncol 2014; 110(2):107–14.

59. Nelson DB, Mehran RJ, Mitchell KG, et al. Enhanced recovery after thoracic surgery is associated with improved adjuvant chemotherapy completion for non-small cell lung cancer. J Thorac Cardiovasc Surg 2019;158(1):279–86.e1.

60. Maruyama R, Miyake T, Kojo M, et al. Establishment of a clinical pathway as an effective tool to reduce hospitalization and charges after video-assisted thoracoscopic pulmonary resection. Jpn J Thorac Cardiovasc Surg 2006;54(9):387–90.

61. Zehr KJ, Dawson PB, Yang SC, et al. Standardized clinical care pathways for major thoracic cases reduce hospital costs. Ann Thorac Surg 1998; 66(3):914–9.

62. Wright CD, Wain JC, Grillo HC, et al. Pulmonary lobectomy patient care pathway: a model to control cost and maintain quality. Ann Thorac Surg 1997; 64(2):299–302.

63. Fiore JF Jr, Bejjani J, Conrad K, et al. Systematic review of the influence of enhanced recovery pathways in elective lung resection. J Thorac Cardiovasc Surg 2016;151(3):708–15.e6.

Open, Minimally Invasive, and Robotic Approaches for Esophagectomy
What Is the Approach Algorithm?

Tadeusz D. Witek, MD[a],*, Thomas J. Melvin, MD[b], James D. Luketich, MD[c],
Inderpal S. Sarkaria, MD, MBA[d]

KEYWORDS

- Esophagectomy • Minimally invasive esophagectomy • Robotic assisted esophagectomy
- Esophageal cancer

KEY POINTS

- Minimally invasive esophagectomy has been described. Regardless of the approach, it is imperative to perform a safe and oncologically sound resection.
- It is important to have a general awareness of risks and advantages of each approach to esophagectomy.
- When it comes to the different approaches to esophagectomy, minimally invasive operations are seen to offer several advantages.
- Several factors can influence the optimal approach; however, the choice of approach largely depends on surgeon comfort and experience.

INTRODUCTION

Esophageal cancer has seen an overall increase in incidence over the last several decades. This pattern is more pronounced in the United States and other Western countries.[1,2] Currently, the incidence of esophageal cancer in the United States approaches 17,000 per year, with more than 15,000 deaths per year attributed to esophageal cancer. It is the eighth most common cancer worldwide, the eighteenth most common in the United States, and only second to pancreatic cancer in case fatality rate.[3,4] The treatment of esophageal cancer revolves around a complex, multimodality approach in most instances, with surgical resection a key component in appropriate patients. With the use of ever improving multimodality therapy, there has been an improvement in long-term survival for those with early or locally advanced disease.[5] This has partly been due to newer chemotherapy agents with lower toxicity profiles, as well as advanced radiotherapy techniques that have developed over the last several decades. Similarly, as other aspects of esophageal cancer treatment have evolved, so has the surgical approach to esophagectomy. Historically, open esophagectomy (OE) by either a transhiatal or transthoracic route has long been the surgical approach to resection; however, over the past several decades, minimally invasive approaches have become more popular, with a greater move

[a] University of Pittsburgh Medical Center, University of Pittsburgh School of Medicine, 200 Lothrop Street, Suite C-800, Pittsburgh, PA 15213, USA; [b] Department of Surgery, University of Pittsburgh Medical Center-Mercy Hospital, UPMC Mercy, 1400 Locust Street, Pittsburgh, PA 15219, USA; [c] University of Pittsburgh Medical Center, University of Pittsburgh School of Medicine, 200 Lothrop Street, Suite C-816, Pittsburgh, PA 15213, USA; [d] University of Pittsburgh Medical Center, University of Pittsburgh School of Medicine, Shadyside Medical Building, 5200 Centre Avenue, Suite 715, Pittsburgh, PA 15232, USA
* Corresponding author.
E-mail address: witektd@upmc.edu

Thorac Surg Clin 30 (2020) 269–277
https://doi.org/10.1016/j.thorsurg.2020.04.010
1547-4127/20/© 2020 Elsevier Inc. All rights reserved.

toward transthoracic rather than transhiatal routes of resection. Regardless of the approach, the goal should remain the same, that is, performing a safe operation without compromise of oncologic principles. Here we discuss the different approaches and variables that may influence decision making.

OPERATIVE APPROACHES

Generally, esophageal resections can be characterized under 2 broad categorizations: transhiatal esophagectomy (THE) versus transthoracic esophagectomy (TTE), and OE versus minimally invasive esophagectomy (MIE). Within these 2 broad categories, subsets of technique exist.

The most common transthoracic operations, those using some component of entry into the right or left lateral chest, include the Ivor Lewis (abdomen and right chest),[6] McKeown or 3-hole (right chest, abdomen, and neck),[7] and right or left (Sweet operation) thoracoabdominal (simultaneous transcostal abdomen and right or left chest).[8] The transhiatal operations are performed through a laparotomy in conjunction with a cervical incision.

Over the last several decades, minimally invasive approaches to esophageal resection have evolved. These approaches were developed to decrease perioperative morbidity, but without compromising oncologic principles. Initially, minimally invasive approaches were used in a limited capacity for small, early stage tumors. With advancements, MIE is often used in advanced cancers as well.[9] MIE includes a large spectrum of approaches. These range from total thoracoscopic and laparoscopic approaches to a variety of hybrid approaches in which the chest approach may be done through a minimally invasive technique, but the abdominal portion remains open, or vice versa. In recent years, robotic approaches to esophagectomy are becoming more popular. Like other MIE approaches, the robot is used either during the chest or abdominal portion, or can be used during the entirety of the resection.

There are a few variables that need to be considered when choosing the approach to surgery for these patients. Ultimately, when resection is performed for malignancy, preserving oncologic principles is key. Regarding robotic resection, the literature continues to expand. Several studies have demonstrated the feasibility of a complete resection.[10–13] In the ROBOT trial, which represents a randomized controlled trial comparing robotic-assisted MIE (RAMIE) with other traditional approaches, R0 resections were comparable between RAMIE and OE, as well as median lymph nodes retrieved.[14] No difference in overall survival

was noted between the 2 groups at 40 months, although longer follow-up will be needed to draw any significant differences.

OPEN VERSUS MINIMALLY INVASIVE ESOPHAGECTOMY

Minimally invasive surgical approaches have been adopted across a wide range of surgical subspecialties. As more physicians became proficient in minimally invasive techniques, several esophageal diseases have been treated in this manner over the past 20 to 30 years; thus, it is no surprise that this has been extended to esophagectomy. As mentioned, the esophagectomy was historically performed in an open fashion, either through the transhiatal or transthoracic approach. However, there are now data that show that these can all be safely performed minimally invasively.[9,15,16] Regardless of the technique or approach used, it is important for the surgeon to be aware of current data regarding morbidity, mortality, and outcomes. Although this area of research is still active area, there is a growing body of literature outlining these techniques.

The morbidity of the OE can exceed 50% to 70%, with mortality historically ranging from 8% to 23%.[9,15,17] However, with the advent of high-volume centers of excellence as well as minimally invasive approaches, these numbers seem to be improving. The literature has substantially grown since the first MIE described by Cuschieri and colleagues[18] in 1992. There are now several randomized trials and meta-analyses that show decreased overall morbidity (especially respiratory complications) and shorter hospital stay for MIE, with similar mortality rates.[9,17,19,20] Anastomotic leakage is an important postoperative morbidity that deserves extra attention. Multiple studies have failed to show a significant difference between open and MIE approaches.[9,15,17,19] In regards to anastomotic technique, stapled anastomosis has been shown to be superior to handsewn techniques in several studies.[21,22] Although this area of research is still active, it seems MIE has several advantages over the traditional open techniques in terms of short-term morbidity.

TRANSTHORACIC VERSUS TRANSHIATAL ESOPHAGECTOMY

When examining the different approaches to esophagectomy, they can broadly be grouped into either TTE or THE, with TTE being subdivided into Ivor Lewis or McKeown methods. In a randomized controlled trial by Omloo and colleagues,[23] the TTE was noted to be superior in several aspects, but primarily better lymph node harvest. This finding has been further validated by several other studies and a large meta-analysis.[9,19,20] Additionally, the TTE has been shown to have a lower anastomotic leak rate when compared with THE.[24] In terms of overall morbidity, THE may be superior. The study from Omloo and colleagues shows less overall morbidity and operative time when the THE approach was used, although this finding has not been routinely replicated in other studies. In a large series by Orringer and colleagues,[25] THE was performed with acceptable morbidity, although anastomotic leak and recurrent laryngeal nerve paralysis was higher compared with those generally reported for Ivor Lewis esophagectomy. The mortality rate of the 2 approaches, however, is largely the same.[9,15–17,26]

As mentioned elsewhere in this article, there are a myriad of surgical approaches to the esophagectomy, and the majority of these can be performed minimally invasively. When comparing the different types of minimally invasive approaches, the transthoracic approaches are subdivided into Ivor Lewis (MIE chest) and McKeown (MIE neck). Although the transhiatal approach can be performed laparoscopically, it is often cited as having poor visibility, often leading to inadequate lymph node dissection and difficulty with hemostasis.[27] Thus, many high-volume centers have transitioned to the transthoracic MIE. The literature comparing the MIE chest and MIE neck is scant. However, a study performed by Luketich and colleagues[9] showed decreased recurrent laryngeal nerve injury and pharyngeal dysfunction in the MIE chest group, with the remaining parameters being similar. Last, robotic approaches have been increasingly used for esophagectomy. Although there is a relative paucity of data regarding its usefulness, several studies show promising results. Early reports have shown RAMIE to offer outcomes similar to other traditional MIE approaches.[11,28,29] Additionally, it is theorized that some areas of the dissection, especially the mediastinum, may be more effectively performed with the robotic platform, given is superior optics, depth of field, and multiple degrees of freedom.[11] However, although promising, this approach needs to be further vetted.

LOCATION

Esophageal cancer may arise anywhere along the esophagus. Squamous cell cancers more commonly occurs in the proximal and middle esophagus, and adenocarcinomas arise in the mid to distal esophagus. To achieve complete (R0) resections, more proximal tumors traditionally require a cervical anastomosis. This goal can be accomplished through either a 3-hole McKeown or transhiatal approach. Either approach can also be accomplished using minimally invasive techniques. As described elsewhere in this article, cervical anastomosis does have a higher incidence of recurrent laryngeal nerve injury, anastomotic leak, and pharyngoesophageal swallowing dysfunction.

When resecting middle to distal esophageal cancers, any esophagectomy technique and approach, open or minimally invasive, can generally be used and performed. We generally recommend an Ivor Lewis approach because it minimizes the risks associated with cervical anastomosis and provides a superior en bloc lymph node resection. Whether it be open or minimally invasive often depends on the surgeon's experience and preference.

PATHOLOGY
Barrett's Esophagus and Malignancy

Historically, Barrett's esophagus (BE) with high-grade dysplasia was an indication for esophageal resection. Today, high-grade dysplasia is frequently treated with endoscopic mucosal resection and ablation of the BE. Indications for esophagectomy in the setting of BE may include multifocal high-grade dysplasia, long segment BE, and a younger patient who may prefer to avoid routine BE surveillance with endoscopic biopsies. Shared decision making between the surgeon and patient would dictate the management in these cases, and a THE with avoidance of the chest and possible pulmonary complications may be offered. Regardless, we prefer to offer a minimally invasive Ivor Lewis approach in these cases to minimize risks of a cervical anastomosis and of laparotomy, including intraoperative cardiac compression, higher splenectomy rate, and long-term risk of ventral hernia.

For locally or regionally advanced esophageal malignancies, the goal is an R0 resection and adequate lymph node harvest for pathologic staging. Histology itself does not directly dictate the approach, but rather the likelihood of a sound oncologic resection. Stage of cancer may impact the surgeon's selection of approach. **Fig. 1** summarizes preferred surgical approaches for esophagectomy in the setting of esophageal malignancy.

Benign Disease

Although less common, occasionally an esophagectomy is warranted for benign disease. Diagnoses include severe refractory reflux disease, end-stage achalasia, severe esophageal dysmotility, and/or stricture. The approach to

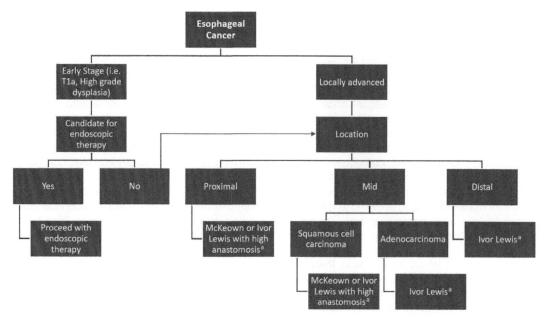

Fig. 1. Surgical approaches to esophagectomy in setting of esophageal malignancy. [a] Choicce of MIE is always preferred, but should be based on experience and comfort level of the surgeon. An open approach should be highly considered if the surgeon is not familiar or experienced with minimally invasive approaches. Strong consideration should be given to minimally invasive approaches for frail patients. Otherwise, a transhiatal or nonoperative approach should be considered.

esophagectomy should be dictated by the disease process. Patients with achalasia or esophageal dysmotility may require a cervical anastomosis to remove all the diseased esophagus. In those undergoing resections for reflux, an Ivor Lewis approach is preferred to avoid complications associated with neck anastomosis. Many patients undergoing esophagectomy for benign pathology have previously undergone one or several prior foregut operations. These may include an antireflux or paraesophageal hernia repair or a modified Heller myotomy. Previous procedures may influence the approach as a completely minimally invasive approach may be impeded by significant scar tissue. In addition, the gastric conduit may no longer be an option after several complex reoperations.[30] Esophagectomy after prior reflux studies has been shown to be associated with greater perioperative morbidity, anastomotic leak, and need for reoperation[31]; however, Chang and colleagues[30] did not report a difference in occurrence of anastomotic leak. **Fig. 2** summarizes preferred surgical approaches for esophagectomy in the setting of benign disease.

LYMPH NODE RESECTION

Although the extent of lymphadenectomy has been an area of controversy for years, several studies have demonstrated that long-term survival may be directly related to this parameter.[32] Hulscher and colleagues[32] have shown an improved lymph node resection through a transthoracic approach, and suggested a survival advantage with improved lyphadencectomy. This outcome is likely from better exposure and improved node dissection in the mediastinum. With regard to open versus minimally invasive transthoracic approach, Luketich and colleagues[9] reported a comparable number of median lymph nodes removed. Other larger studies have reported similar findings.[33,34] Ye and colleagues[35] have reported an increased extent of lymphadenectomy in higher stage squamous cell carcinoma. As far as RAMIE approaches, several series have demonstrated an improved lymph node resection compared with an open approach.[14,28,36–38]

ONCOLOGIC OUTCOMES

For OE, studies have not routinely shown significant differences in long-term survival between transhiatal and transthoracic approches.[39,40] In a large randomized study by Hulscher and colleagues[32] comparing TTE and THE, R0 resection was similar. Significantly more lymph nodes were resected in the TTE arm. The recurrence rate and

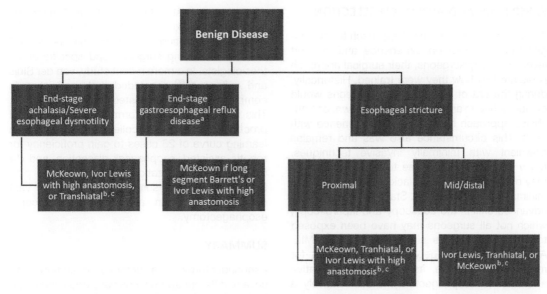

Fig. 2. Surgical approaches to esophagectomy in setting of benign disease. [a] Patients with multiple failed anti-reflux surgeries that are not amendable to redo fundoplication or Roux-en-Y. [b] Choice of MIE is always preferred, but should be based on experience and comfort level of the surgeon. An open approach should be highly considered if the surgeon is not familiar or experienced with minimally invasive approaches. Strong consideration should be given to minimally invasive approaches for frail patients. [c] If unable to perform a minimally invasive procedure, a transhiatal approach would be preferred to avoid morbidity associated with a thoracotomy.

median disease-free survival were similar. There was a trend toward a better 5-year survival in the TTE group, but it was not statistically significant.

Many series have shown MIE to be oncologically comparable with OE.[41] In a meta-analysis performed by Gottlieb-Vedi and colleagues,[42] long-term survival after MIE was similar and potentially even be better than OE. As far as adequacy of resection, in one of the largest series to date on MIE, Luketich and colleagues[9] reported an R0 resection in 98% of patients.[9] Lymph node resection, as mentioned elsewhere in this article, is similar to open approach.[33,34] In patients who underwent neoadjuvant therapy, MIE approaches are equivalent to open approaches in regard to perioperative outcomes.[43]

There are few data on long-term cancer survival after RAMIE. As far as adequacy of resection, Puntambekar and associates[44] reported a 97.6% R0 resection with a hybrid robotic-assisted 3-hole esophagectomy. As for the Ivor Lewis RAMIE, several series have reported a complete resection from 90% to 100%.[10–13] Although the ROBOT trial, a randomized controlled trial comparing a robotic versus a traditional approach, did not focus on survival outcomes, several oncologic outcomes were extrapolated. R0 resections were comparable

between RAMIE and OE (93% vs 96%; P = .35). At median follow-up of 40 months, overall survival and disease-free survival were not statistically significantly different between the RAMIE and OE arms.[14] Recurrence rates in this series were also consistent with published data on OE.[45] As mentioned elsewhere in this article, several studies have reported an improved lymph node resection compared with an open approach.[14,28,36,37,46] Increased lymph node resection may potentially offer some benefit in regard to overall cancer survival, although further studies would need to be completed to confirm any oncologic advantage.

QUALITY OF LIFE

Improved quality of life after esophagectomy can be a predictor of long-term survival.[47,48] Global health, social, and emotional functioning improve more frequently after MIE compared with OE.[49] In a randomized study from the Netherlands, MIE was associated with better quality of life at 1 year after resection.[50] In the ROBOT trial, compared with OE, the RAMIE arm had improved functional recovery at 14 days, less postoperative pain, and overall better quality of life based on assessment tools.[14] Other studies also reported less pain after RAMIE.[46,51]

EXPERIENCE AND APPROACH SELECTION

A large influence on surgical approach to esophagectomy is based on experience and comfort level. For many surgeons, their surgical approach is dictated by how they were trained. Historically, during the era of open surgery, surgeons would decide between an Ivor Lewis, McKeown, or transhiatal approach based on their experience with each. This circumstance also was and remains prevalent with minimally invasive techniques. Many surgeons still choose to do an OE, which may often be due to their lack of experience with minimally invasive surgery. Standard MIE requires advanced skill in thoracoscopy and laparoscopy, which not all surgeons may have been exposed to in training. This is also the case in RAMIE. Although robotic surgery has been present for more than a decade, its use as an alternative approach to esophagectomy is still relatively a younger adaptation.

Previous studies have evaluated the learning curve in regards to MIE. Guo and colleagues[52] reported that 30 cases were needed to gain proficiency, with even lower morbidity at 60 cases. Other studies reported similar findings.[53] Although earlier studies focused on parameters directly related to the surgery, specifically operative time, more recent studies evaluated the effects of the learning curve on anastomotic leakage, mortality, and survival. Van Workum and colleagues[54] reported that 10% of leaks were attributed to the learning curve phase. Several studies also identified increased mortality associated with learning curve.[55,56] These findings stress the importance of rigid structured training and proctorship when first endeavoring in MIE.

When it comes robotics, some investigators argue that the learning curve is decreased compared with standard minimally invasive approach owing to the sophistication of the robotic technology.[11,57] Several studies have attempted to define proficiency in robotic esophagectomies. Hernandez and cowrokers[58] reported near proficiency around 20 cases, at which point operative time was significantly decreased. Other studies also noted that proficiency was can be achieved early on.[44,59] It is important to note, however, that obtaining proficiency has many variables, including previous experience in esophagectomy and robotic surgery. Also, the extent of the robotic portion of the esophagectomy may vary between studies. In a study by Sarkaria and colleagues[13] regarding learning curve in completely robotic RAMIE, significant decrease in operative times were noted between 30 and 45 cases with the nadir between cases 40 and 45. Conversion rates decreased from 13 in the first 50 to 2 in the next 50 cases. The study ensured a dedicated operating room team that included 2 constant attending surgeons and specific anesthesiologists. In a more recent study, van der Sluis and colleagues[60] concluded that proficiency in completely RAMIE consisted of 70 procedures. This study was also performed under structured proctoring. Zhang and colleagues[61] reported a learning curve of 26 cases to gain proficiency for robotic-assisted esophageal dissection and 14 for stomach mobilization. This study was performed by a single surgical team that had vast experience in open and thoracolaparoscopic esophagectomy.

SUMMARY

Esophagectomy is a complex operation, and several different approaches have been historically described. The major approaches include transhiatal or transthoracic, with the latter being primarily subdivided into the Ivor Lewis, McKeown, and thoracoabdominal operations. All of these procedures can be performed minimally invasively, and with or without robotic assistance. Although minimally invasive operations may offer several advantages in the perioperative period, the decision to perform an open or minimally operation must be tempered primarily by surgeon comfort and experience with any given approach. Regardless of which approach is chosen, it is paramount to focus primarily on a safe and oncologically sound resection.

DISCLOSURE

The authors have nothing to disclose.

REFERENCES

1. Blot WJ, McLaughlin JK. The changing epidemiology of esophageal cancer. Semin Oncol 1999; 26(5 Suppl 15):2–8.
2. Pohl H, Welch HG. The role of overdiagnosis and reclassification in the marked increase of esophageal adenocarcinoma incidence. J Natl Cancer Inst 2005;97(2):142–6.
3. Ferlay J, Soerjomataram I, Dikshit R, et al. Cancer incidence and mortality worldwide: sources, methods and major patterns in GLOBOCAN 2012. Int J Cancer 2015;136(5):E359–86.
4. Siegel RL, Miller KD, Jemal A. Cancer statistics, 2015. CA Cancer J Clin 2015;65(1):5–29.
5. Rustgi AK, El-Serag HB. Esophageal carcinoma. N Engl J Med 2014;371(26):2499–509.
6. Lewis I. The surgical treatment of carcinoma of the oesophagus; with special reference to a new

operation for growths of the middle third. Br J Surg 1946;34:18–31.

7. McKeown KC. Total three-stage oesophagectomy for cancer of the oesophagus. Br J Surg 1976; 63(4):259–62.

8. Sweet RH. Carcinoma of the esophagus and the cardiac end of the stomach immediate and late results of treatment by resection and primary esophagogastric anastomosis. J Am Med Assoc 1947; 135(8):485–90.

9. Luketich JD, Pennathur A, Awais O, et al. Outcomes after minimally invasive esophagectomy: review of over 1000 patients. Ann Surg 2012;256(1):95–103.

10. Hodari A, Park KU, Lace B, et al. Robot-assisted minimally invasive Ivor Lewis esophagectomy with real-time perfusion assessment. Ann Thorac Surg 2015;100(3):947–52.

11. Okusanya OT, Sarkaria IS, Hess NR, et al. Robotic assisted minimally invasive esophagectomy (RAMIE): the University of Pittsburgh Medical Center initial experience. Ann Cardiothorac Surg 2017;6(2): 179–85.

12. Sarkaria IS, Rizk NP. Robotic-assisted minimally invasive esophagectomy: the Ivor Lewis approach. Thorac Surg Clin 2014;24(2):211–22, vii.

13. Sarkaria IS, Rizk NP, Grosser R, et al. Attaining proficiency in robotic-assisted minimally invasive esophagectomy while maximizing safety during procedure development. Innovations (Phila) 2016; 11(4):268–73.

14. van der Sluis PC, van der Horst S, May AM, et al. Robot-assisted minimally invasive thoracolaparoscopic esophagectomy versus open transthoracic esophagectomy for resectable esophageal cancer: a randomized controlled trial. Ann Surg 2019; 269(4):621–30.

15. Levy RM, Trivedi D, Luketich JD. Minimally invasive esophagectomy. Surg Clin North Am 2012;92(5): 1265–85.

16. van den Berg JW, Luketich JD, Cheong E. Oesophagectomy: the expanding role of minimally invasive surgery in oesophageal cancer. Best Pract Res Clin Gastroenterol 2018;36-37:75–80.

17. Levy RM, Pennathur A, Luketich JD. Randomized trial comparing minimally invasive esophagectomy and open esophagectomy: early perioperative outcomes appear improved with a minimally invasive approach. Semin Thorac Cardiovasc Surg 2012; 24(3):153–4.

18. Cuschieri A, Shimi S, Banting S. Endoscopic oesophagectomy through a right thoracoscopic approach. J R Coll Surg Edinb 1992;37(1):7–11.

19. Biere SS, van Berge Henegouwen MI, Maas KW, et al. Minimally invasive versus open oesophagectomy for patients with oesophageal cancer: a multicentre, open-label, randomised controlled trial. Lancet 2012;379(9829):1887–92.

20. Heger P, Blank S, Goossen K, et al. Thoracoabdominal versus transhiatal surgical approaches for adenocarcinoma of the esophagogastric junction-a systematic review and meta-analysis. Langenbecks Arch Surg 2019;404(1):103–13.

21. Kumar T, Krishanappa R, Pai E, et al. Completely linear stapled versus handsewn cervical esophagogastric anastomosis after esophagectomy. Indian J Surg 2018;80(2):134–9.

22. Pines G, Buyeviz V, Machlenkin S, et al. The use of circular stapler for cervical esophagogastric anastomosis after esophagectomy: surgical technique and early postoperative outcome. Dis Esophagus 2009; 22(3):274–8.

23. Omloo JM, Lagarde SM, Hulscher JB, et al. Extended transthoracic resection compared with limited transhiatal resection for adenocarcinoma of the mid/distal esophagus: five-year survival of a randomized clinical trial. Ann Surg 2007;246(6): 992–1000 [discussion: 1000–1].

24. Ryan CE, Paniccia A, Meguid RA, et al. Transthoracic anastomotic leak after esophagectomy: current trends. Ann Surg Oncol 2017;24(1): 281–90.

25. Orringer MB, Marshall B, Iannettoni MD. Transhiatal esophagectomy: clinical experience and refinements. Ann Surg 1999;230(3):392–400 [discussion: 400–3].

26. Biere SS, van Berge Henegouwen MI, Bonavina L, et al. Predictive factors for post-operative respiratory infections after esophagectomy for esophageal cancer: outcome of randomized trial. J Thorac Dis 2017; 9(Suppl 8):S861–7.

27. Levy RM, Wizorek J, Shende M, et al. Laparoscopic and thoracoscopic esophagectomy. Adv Surg 2010; 44:101–16.

28. Meredith KL, Maramara T, Blinn P, et al. Comparative perioperative outcomes by esophagectomy surgical technique. J Gastrointest Surg 2019. [Epub ahead of print].

29. van der Sluis PC, van Hillegersberg R. Robot assisted minimally invasive esophagectomy (RAMIE) for esophageal cancer. Best Pract Res Clin Gastroenterol 2018;36-37:81–3.

30. Chang AC, Lee JS, Sawicki KT, et al. Outcomes after esophagectomy in patients with prior antireflux or hiatal hernia surgery. Ann Thorac Surg 2010;89(4): 1015–21 [discussion: 1022–3].

31. Shen KR, Harrison-Phipps KM, Cassivi SD, et al. Esophagectomy after anti-reflux surgery. J Thorac Cardiovasc Surg 2010;139(4):969–75.

32. Hulscher JB, van Sandick JW, de Boer AG, et al. Extended transthoracic resection compared with limited transhiatal resection for adenocarcinoma of the esophagus. N Engl J Med 2002;347(21): 1662–9.

33. Seesing MFJ, Gisbertz SS, Goense L, et al. A propensity score matched analysis of open

versus minimally invasive transthoracic esopha-gectomy in the Netherlands. Ann Surg 2017; 266(5):839–46.

34. Yibulayin W, Abulizi S, Lv H, et al. Minimally invasive oesophagectomy versus open esophagectomy for resectable esophageal cancer: a meta-analysis. World J Surg Oncol 2016;14(1):304.

35. Ye B, Zhong CX, Yang Y, et al. Lymph node dissection in esophageal carcinoma: minimally invasive esophagectomy vs open surgery. World J Gastroenterol 2016;22(19):4750–6.

36. Espinoza-Mercado F, Imai TA, Borgella JD, et al. Does the approach matter? Comparing survival in robotic, minimally invasive, and open esophagectomies. Ann Thorac Surg 2019;107(2):378–85.

37. Mori K, Yamagata Y, Aikou S, et al. Short-term outcomes of robotic radical esophagectomy for esophageal cancer by a nontransthoracic approach compared with conventional transthoracic surgery. Dis Esophagus 2016;29(5):429–34.

38. Sarkaria IS, Rizk NP, Finley DJ, et al. Combined thoracoscopic and laparoscopic robotic-assisted minimally invasive esophagectomy using a four-arm platform: experience, technique and cautions during early procedure development. Eur J Cardiothorac Surg 2013;43(5):e107–15.

39. Hulscher JB, Tijssen JG, Obertop H, et al. Transthoracic versus transhiatal resection for carcinoma of the esophagus: a meta-analysis. Ann Thorac Surg 2001;72(1):306–13.

40. Rindani R, Martin CJ, Cox MR. Transhiatal versus Ivor-Lewis oesophagectomy: is there a difference? Aust N Z J Surg 1999;69(3):187–94.

41. Verhage RJ, Hazebroek EJ, Boone J, et al. Minimally invasive surgery compared to open procedures in esophagectomy for cancer: a systematic review of the literature. Minerva Chir 2009;64(2):135–46.

42. Gottlieb-Vedi E, Kauppila JH, Malietzis G, et al. Long-term survival in esophageal cancer after minimally invasive compared to open esophagectomy: a systematic review and meta-analysis. Ann Surg 2019;270(6):1005–17.

43. Tapias LF, Mathisen DJ, Wright CD, et al. Outcomes with open and minimally invasive Ivor Lewis esophagectomy after neoadjuvant therapy. Ann Thorac Surg 2016;101(3):1097–103.

44. Puntambekar S, Kenawadekar R, Kumar S, et al. Robotic transthoracic esophagectomy. BMC Surg 2015;15:47.

45. van Hagen P, Wijnhoven BP, Nafteux P, et al. Recurrence pattern in patients with a pathologically complete response after neoadjuvant chemoradiotherapy and surgery for oesophageal cancer. Br J Surg 2013; 100(2):267–73.

46. Sarkaria IS, Rizk NP, Goldman DA, et al. Early quality of life outcomes after robotic-assisted minimally invasive and open esophagectomy. Ann Thorac Surg 2019;108(3):920–8.

47. Safieddine N, Xu W, Quadri SM, et al. Health-related quality of life in esophageal cancer: effect of neoadjuvant chemoradiotherapy followed by surgical intervention. J Thorac Cardiovasc Surg 2009;137(1): 36–42.

48. van Heijl M, Sprangers MA, de Boer AG, et al. Preoperative and early postoperative quality of life predict survival in potentially curable patients with esophageal cancer. Ann Surg Oncol 2010;17(1): 23–30.

49. Taioli E, Schwartz RM, Lieberman-Cribbin W, et al. Quality of life after open or minimally invasive esophagectomy in patients with esophageal cancer-a systematic review. Semin Thorac Cardiovasc Surg 2017;29(3):377–90.

50. Maas KW, Cuesta MA, van Berge Henegouwen MI, et al. Quality of life and late complications after minimally invasive compared to open esophagectomy: results of a randomized trial. World J Surg 2015; 39(8):1986–93.

51. Sugawara K, Yoshimura S, Yagi K, et al. Long-term health-related quality of life following robot-assisted radical transmediastinal esophagectomy. Surg Endosc 2020;34(4):1602–11.

52. Guo W, Zou YB, Ma Z, et al. One surgeon's learning curve for video-assisted thoracoscopic esophagectomy for esophageal cancer with the patient in lateral position: how many cases are needed to reach competence? Surg Endosc 2013;27(4): 1346–52.

53. Lin J, Kang M, Chen C, et al. Thoracolaparoscopy oesophagectomy and extensive two-field lymphadenectomy for oesophageal cancer: introduction and teaching of a new technique in a high-volume centre. Eur J Cardiothorac Surg 2013;43(1): 115–21.

54. van Workum F, Stenstra M, Berkelmans GHK, et al. Learning curve and associated morbidity of minimally invasive esophagectomy: a retrospective multicenter study. Ann Surg 2019;269(1):88–94.

55. Mackenzie H, Markar SR, Askari A, et al. National proficiency-gain curves for minimally invasive gastrointestinal cancer surgery. Br J Surg 2016; 103(1):88–96.

56. Markar SR, Mackenzie H, Lagergren P, et al. Surgical proficiency gain and survival after esophagectomy for cancer. J Clin Oncol 2016;34(13): 1528–36.

57. Kumar A, Asaf BB. Robotic thoracic surgery: the state of the art. J Minim Access Surg 2015;11(1): 60–7.

58. Hernandez JM, Dimou F, Weber J, et al. Defining the learning curve for robotic-assisted esophagogastrectomy. J Gastrointest Surg 2013;17(8):1346–51.

59. Kim DJ, Hyung WJ, Lee CY, et al. Thoracoscopic esophagectomy for esophageal cancer: feasibility and safety of robotic assistance in the prone position. J Thorac Cardiovasc Surg 2010;139(1): 53–9.e51.

60. van der Sluis PC, Ruurda JP, van der Horst S, et al. Learning curve for robot-assisted minimally invasive thoracoscopic esophagectomy: results from 312 cases. Ann Thorac Surg 2018;106(1): 264–71.

61. Zhang H, Chen L, Wang Z, et al. The learning curve for robotic McKeown esophagectomy in patients with esophageal cancer. Ann Thorac Surg 2018; 105(4):1024–30.

Section B: Intraoperative management

Intraoperative Anesthetic Management of the Thoracic Patient

Melina Shoni, MD[a], Gerardo Rodriguez, MD[b],*

KEYWORDS

- One-lung ventilation complications • Double-lumen endobronchial tube • Bronchial blocker
- Hypoxic pulmonary vasoconstriction • Hypoxemia and one-lung ventilation

KEY POINTS

- Serious complications from one-lung ventilation include arterial hypoxemia, injury to the nonoperative lung, and right ventricular dysfunction.
- Understanding the effects of anesthetic agents on hypoxic pulmonary vasoconstriction is important for optimizing oxygenation during thoracic surgery.
- Individualized one-lung ventilation management strategies, influenced by the patient's risk for developing hypoxemia, the surgical approach, and the airway device selected, can improve postoperative outcomes.
- Goal-directed fluid therapy and perioperative pain management strategies can reduce morbidity after thoracic surgery.

INTRODUCTION

The concept of lung isolation dates back to the 1870s when experimental physiologists Edward Pflüger and Claude Bernard introduced the first example of a single-lumen endobronchial cannula.[1] The transition from single-lumen endobronchial cannulas to double-lumen cannulas that combined short-tracheal and long-bronchial segments in 1889 facilitated many advances in respiratory physiology and independent lung spirometry.[1] Over the years, these techniques led to a practical progression in human airway instrumentation devices, including two-cuff single-lumen endobronchial tubes (SLTs), double-lumen endobronchial tubes (DLTs), and bronchial blockers (BBs). This specialized armamentarium established the anesthetic practice of one-lung ventilation (OLV) and enabled the performance of complex lung, esophageal, mediastinal, and thoracic wall operations.

ONE-LUNG VENTILATION

OLV can be defined as the preferential ventilation of the nonoperative lung while deflating the operative lung to achieve an immobile surgical field and to prevent surgical debris, pus, or secretions from entering the contralateral lung (**Box 1**). The extent of lung deflation differentiates lung separation (adequate deflation) from lung isolation (complete deflation).[2] In routine practice, OLV is initiated intraoperatively by the anesthesiologist when the surgeon communicates that the pleura is opened; however, there is evidence to support preemptive OLV immediately after lateral positioning for expedited lung collapse.[3]

Double-Lumen Endobronchial Tubes

The modern version of the DLT stems from a breakthrough invention in 1949 by the Swedish

---

Funding: None.
[a] Department of Anesthesiology, Boston Medical Center, 750 Albany Street, Power Plant, 2nd Floor, Boston, MA 02118, USA; [b] Surgical Intensive Care Unit, Department of Anesthesiology, Boston University School of Medicine, Boston Medical Center, 750 Albany Street, Power Plant, 2nd Floor, Boston, MA 02118, USA
* Corresponding author.
E-mail address: gerardo.rodriguez@bmc.org

Thorac Surg Clin 30 (2020) 279–291
https://doi.org/10.1016/j.thorsurg.2020.04.011

Box 1
Common indications for one-lung ventilation

Surgical exposure

- Pulmonary resection
- Video-assisted thoracoscopic surgery
- Thoracoscopy
- Lung biopsy
- Lymph node biopsy
- Thoracic aortic surgery
- Esophageal surgery
- Mediastinal surgery
- Thoracic wall surgery

Protective lung isolation

- Malignancy
- Purulent material
- Massive hemoptysis

Differential lung ventilation

- Single-lung transplant
- Bronchopleural fistula
- Bronchial disruption
- Asymmetric parenchymal lung disease

Unilateral bronchial lavage

- Pulmonary alveolar proteinosis

physician Eric Carlens.[4] He advanced a red rubber tube with a cuff down to the left main bronchus to seal off the left lung. The tube had a carinal hook to stabilize against the carina. Above the carinal hook was an opening for ventilation of the right main bronchus. Proximal to this was the tracheal cuff. In 1962, Robertshaw[5] refined Carlen's design by eliminating the carinal hook, widening the D-shaped lumens to lower airflow resistance and facilitate suctioning, and incorporating a flatter extrusion to make it more stable and easier to handle. He designed both left-sided (angle of 45° at the carina) and right-sided (angle of 20° at the carina) DLTs.

Today's DLTs are the preferred device for OLV with the longest track record in clinical practice.[6] The consistent and more convenient design of left DLTs among manufacturers has led to their domination compared with the right DLTs. A DLT that is appropriately sized and placed is key to preventing airway injury and achieving proper lung isolation. The optimal DLT size is considered the largest size that will pass uneventfully through

the glottis and trachea and whose bronchial component sits in the mainstem bronchus with only a small air leak. Still, appropriate DLT size selection based on patient factors remains controversial. Chest radiography,[7] computed tomography, and ultrasonography (US) to measure patient tracheal diameter have been suggested.[8] Roldi and colleagues[9] combined patient sex and height with US-derived tracheal measurements to predict DLT size. An undersized DLT can increase the risk of auto positive end-expiratory pressure (PEEP) and dynamic pulmonary hyperinflation, bronchial cuff hyperinflation, failed lung collapse, and possibly tube malposition.[10] Fiber-optic bronchoscopy remains the gold standard for confirming DLT placement; blindly placed DLTs can be malpositioned up to 48% of the time.[11]

Bronchial Blockers

The use of a BB for OLV is increasing worldwide. Various BB types are currently available (**Table 1**). The specific features of a BB dictate its utilization. Adult sizes are 9 French. Pediatric sizes are 5 French. **Table 2** provides a comparison between DLTs and BBs. For most patients, the BB is an appropriate option except for operations involving the main bronchus, distorted bronchial anatomy, or bronchopulmonary lavage. Some advantages of BBs over DLTs include use in patients with difficult airway anatomy where DLT placement may be impossible, patients at high risk for aspiration, patients with tracheostomy, children, surgical procedures with a high risk of left recurrent laryngeal nerve injury, or surgeries requiring postoperative mechanical ventilation.[12–14] Overall, the rate of major complications from BBs is low.[15] However, minor airway trauma, failure to achieve lung separation or isolation, balloon malpositioning, device technical malfunctioning (eg, fractured or bent tips, difficult balloon deflation and retrieval, asymmetrical balloon inflation), and inadvertent entrapment of the BB in the surgical staple line have been reported.[16,17]

The debate over which device is best for OLV is still ongoing.[18,19] For most thoracic procedures, either device can be used safely. The choice is usually based on the specific requirements of each case, patient airway anatomy, and the preference and experience of the anesthesiologist. A recent survey in the United Kingdom among anesthesiologists revealed a 98% preference rate for DLT use, and 64% of respondents reported rarely using a BB to provide lung isolation.[20] Although surgeons seem to also prefer DLTs, studies support similar quality in lung isolation between

Table 1
Types of bronchial blockers

Univent Torque Control (Fuji Systems, Tokyo, Japan)	First manufactured BB; contains a single lumen for ventilation and a channel that houses the BB; bulky tube for the size of its ventilating lumen. Out of favor
Cohen Flex-tip (Cook Medical Inc, Bloomington, IN, USA)	Has a wheel at the operator end that, when turned, flexes the tip; advancement of the BB is observed via a fiberscope, which also is passed through a multiport connector
Arndt (Cook Medical Inc, Bloomington, IN, USA)	Has a lumen through which a wire passes and exits in a loop, beyond its distal end. The fiberscope is passed through this loop and is advanced into the mainstem bronchus with the BB trailing. The wires nare is loosened and then is removed once the BB is in place. The position of the BB then is checked as the fiberscope is withdrawn. Somewhat cumbersome to use, with multiple steps needed for proper placement
Uniblocker (Fuji Systems, Tokyo, Japan)	The most newly released, simplest in design and usage. The BB has a bent tip and comes preinserted through a multiport connector. It is simply turned toward the side to be blocked and advanced under direct vision with the fiber-optic bronchoscope. Viable option for those with limited thoracic anesthesia experience, and placement actually may be easier than a DLT. It is also significantly less expensive, although more costly than a DLT
Rusch EZ (Teleflex Medical, Morrisville, NC, USA)	Y-shaped distal end with 1 blocker for each bronchus. Similar quality of lung isolation. Can be placed blindly if a fiberscope is not available or if visualization proves difficult. Lower incidence of airway injury than DLT

DLTs and BBs.[13,21] Successful utilization of BBs relies on the operator's skill and knowledge of airway anatomy, the device itself, and the fiberscope.[13] A systematic review and meta-analysis of 39 randomized controlled trials comparing DLTs and BBs for OLV concluded that DLTs were quicker to place and less likely to be positioned incorrectly, but had a higher complication rate. BBs appeared to have a lower incidence of sore throat, hoarseness, and severe airway injury.[15,22] Thus, for optimal patient care and maintaining technical skills, it is important to develop the skills needed to use both DLTs and BBs.

Two-Cuffed Single-Lumen Endobronchial Tubes

SLTs are another alternative to DLTs and BBs. They have a single lumen with a distal bronchial cuff and a proximal tracheal cuff and are guided either to the right or to the left mainstem bronchus.

Both lungs can be ventilated when the upper cuff is inflated, and the tip of the tube remains in the trachea. When advanced to one of the main bronchi, OLV of the intubated lung is achieved by keeping the upper cuff deflated and the lower one inflated. Despite the efficient design of the SLT, it has fallen out of favor because of an inability to aspirate secretions from the operative lung, as well as the risk of right upper lobe orifice obstruction during right lung ventilation.[2]

COMPLICATIONS OF ONE-LUNG VENTILATION
Hypoxemia

During OLV, the operative lung is excluded from ventilation while it continues to be perfused. This large ventilation-to-perfusion (V/Q) mismatch creates an obligatory intrapulmonary shunt with resultant hypoxemia defined as oxygen saturation (Spo_2) less than 90% or partial pressure of arterial

Table 2
The advantages and disadvantages of double-lumen endobronchial tube and bronchial blocker

	DLT		BB
+ +	Applicable for every thoracic operation Only device suitable for bronchopulmonary lavage	–	Not suitable for thoracic operations that involve the main bronchus (eg, sleeve resection, major bronchopleural fistula, lung transplant, bronchopulmonary lavage, atypical bronchial anatomy)
+	Safe, easy, quick, accurate placement	–	Higher-risk incorrect positioning
+	Both lung separation and isolation	+	Both lung separation and isolation of similar quality with DLTs
+	Rapid lung deflation-reinflation as many times as needed (useful in short procedures)	–	Longer time to achieve lung separation or isolation
+	Less intraoperative displacement/ repositioning	–	Increased risk of balloon displacement with sequential inflation/deflation of the operated lung or patient position changes
+	Suitable for operation in both sides and for sequential surgery to both lungs during the same operation	–	Not recommended
+	Allows suctioning of both lungs without interrupting ventilation	–	Limited options for adequate suctioning without interrupting ventilation or contaminating the contralateral lung
+	Allows bronchoscopy of non–ventilated lung	–	Inability for visual examination of the non–ventilated lung
+	Allows application of CPAP to non–ventilated lung	–	Difficult application of CPAP to non–ventilated lung due to smaller BB lumen
+	Allows differential lung ventilation in ICU	–	Does not allow differential lung ventilation in ICU
+	Inexpensive disposable DLTs	–	More expensive than disposable DLTs
–	Only oral intubation	+	Both nasal and oral intubation
–	No available DLT for tracheostomies	+	Ability to pass through tracheostomies
–	Bulky device	+	Appropriate size to pass via SLT or laryngeal mask airway device
–	Inability to selective lobes or segments	+	Ability to deflate selective lobes or segments
–	Difficulties with endobronchial positioning	+	Easier endobronchial placement
–	Higher risk of airway trauma	+	Lower risk of airway trauma
–	Requires exchange to SLT for patients planned for postoperative ventilation	+	Obviates multiple tube exchanges; particularly useful in cases with difficult airway, airway edema, distorted upper and lower airway anatomy, long surgery, need for continued postoperative mechanical ventilation
–	Higher risk of adverse events	+	Slightly lower risk of adverse events
–	Risky tube exchange for patients already intubated with SLT	+	Safer option for patients already intubated with SLT

oxygen (PaO_2) less than 60 mm Hg. Furthermore, alveolar derecruitment of the nonoperative lung from general anesthesia and lateral positioning also contributes to arterial hypoxemia.[23] Wang and colleagues[24] estimated the shunt fraction after 30 and 60 minutes of OLV to be 35% and 37%, respectively, with an inverse correlation between PaO_2 and V/Q mismatch.

In response, hypoxic pulmonary vasoconstriction (HPV) activates and redirects blood flow from poorly ventilated lung regions, operative lung, to well-ventilated lung regions, nonoperative lung, to decrease the intrapulmonary shunt.[25] Factors that inhibit HPV, such as inhaled anesthetics, hypotension, severe chronic obstructive pulmonary disease (COPD), and use of vasodilators or vasoconstrictors, will divert blood flow to the operative lung and worsen V/Q mismatch and hypoxemia. Factors that improve V/Q matching include lateral decubitus position and moderate COPD with air trapping. The likelihood of a patient developing hypoxemia during OLV is associated with several patient- and surgery-specific risk factors (**Table 3**).[26–29]

Thanks to improved lung isolation devices, improved positioning techniques, and newer anesthetics, the incidence of hypoxemia during OLV has decreased from 25% in the 1970s to 4% to 10% today.[30] Healthy individuals can tolerate hypoxemia during OLV,[31] and SaO_2 as low as 85% to 90% may be acceptable.[31,32] Individuals with coexisting cardiovascular, cerebrovascular, or pulmonary disease, however, are at greater risk for hypoxemia-induced complications, including myocardial depression, atrial fibrillation, pulmonary hypertension, and cognitive dysfunction.[33]

Judicious delivery of oxygen is recommended to maintain adequate oxygenation yet minimize the deleterious effects of hyperoxia, such as inflammation, oxidative stress, alveolar wall thickening, absorption atelectasis, and coronary and peripheral vasoconstriction.[34]

Hypoxemia during OLV can be managed methodically and sequentially. First, the fraction of inspired oxygen (FiO_2) can be increased to 1.0.

An alveolar recruitment maneuver (ARM), consisting of 10 consecutive breaths at a plateau pressure of 40 mm Hg, can be tried next. Notably, a preemptive ARM of both lungs before instituting OLV has been shown to decrease alveolar dead space and improve arterial oxygenation.[35,36] The high plateau pressure associated with an ARM can cause transient hemodynamic derangements and, therefore, should be considered carefully before routine use.[37]

Incremental increases in PEEP to the nonoperative lung to a maximum 20 cm H_2O can be attempted to open atelectatic alveoli.[35,38,39] Careful attention is warranted as PEEP is adjusted. When PEEP causes the end-expiratory pressure to approach the inflection point of the patient's static lung compliance curve, oxygenation is likely to improve. Conversely, if the equilibrium end-expiratory pressure increases beyond the inflection point, oxygenation is likely to deteriorate.[40] The application of PEEP to the nonoperative lung should be individualized by using a PEEP decrement trial; this can improve oxygenation, ventilation, and lung mechanics compared with a standard increase in PEEP of 5 cm H_2O.[41] Clinical trials examining the effect of individualized perioperative ventilator strategies[42] as well high versus low PEEP during OLV are ongoing.[43]

Apneic oxygen insufflation or continuous positive airway pressure (CPAP) to the operative lung should be considered to improve oxygenation by passive mechanics.[44] In the specific cases whereby CPAP may be contraindicated, including video-assisted thoracoscopic surgery, high-frequency jet ventilation to the operative lung has been used to assist with both oxygenation and ventilation, while maintaining an acceptable surgical field of vision.[45] Recently, differential lung ventilation has been described whereby the operative lung is ventilated with minimal tidal volumes (TV).[46]

If hypoxemia persists, two-lung ventilation should be restored to allow for fiber-optic assessment of the lung isolation device position and the presence of secretions. As a last resort, during

Table 3	
Risk factors for developing hypoxemia during one-lung ventilation can be classified as patient specific and surgery specific	
Patient-Specific Risk Factors	**Surgery-Specific Risk Factors**
• Normal preoperative spirometry • Body mass index >30 kg/m^2 • Low baseline PaO_2 • History of lung-reducing operation	• Large, central lung mass • Right-sided thoracic surgery • Surgery performed in the supine position

open thoracotomy, the surgeon can clamp the pulmonary artery (PA) to the operative lung to reduce the shunt fraction and improve oxygenation.

Less common methods for improving refractory oxygenation involve the pharmacologic manipulation of pulmonary blood flow. Total intravenous anesthesia (TIVA) avoids volatile anesthetics and could theoretically preserve HPV, although significant improvements in hypoxemia have not been reported.[47] Selective dilation of the pulmonary vessels in ventilated lung regions with inhaled nitric oxide (iNO)[48] or selective constriction of pulmonary vessels in nonventilated regions with almitrine[49–51] have produced mixed results. Improved oxygenation has been achieved with small doses of iNO[52] in patients with pulmonary hypertension and hypoxemia during OLV.[53] Inhaled iloprost, a prostacyclin analogue, can also improve oxygenation by selectively vasodilating the pulmonary vascular bed and ameliorating V/Q mismatch.[54] The continuous infusion of dexmedetomidine has demonstrated clinical benefits by improving oxygenation and lung mechanics in patients with moderate COPD undergoing lung surgery,[55] which was further supported by a subsequent meta-analysis.[56]

For patients at high risk for developing hypoxemia during OLV, additional monitors can help. Oxygen reverse index is a novel noninvasive continuous monitor of real-time blood oxygenation. Based on multi-wavelength pulse cooximetry, its values correlate strongly with Pao_2 and decrease earlier than Spo_2, identifying hypoxemia earlier.[57–60] Cerebral oxygen saturation ($Scto_2$) can also be monitored, especially in patients at higher risk for postoperative neurocognitive dysfunction. Studies investigating the role of cerebral oximetry in OLV, however, have had mixed results.[61–65] Interestingly, greater decreases in $Scto_2$ during OLV were found in patients with good preoperative respiratory function compared with patients with poor respiratory function. Although reasons for this paradoxic finding remain unknown, it is theorized that chronic lung disease may induce an oxygen reserve enhancement in some patients.[62] More studies are needed to demonstrate the changes in $Scto_2$ during OLV and their association with hypoxemic events measured by Spo_2.

Acute Lung Injury

Acute lung injury (ALI) is characterized by a deleterious cascade of inflammatory and vascular permeability changes within the lung parenchyma that results in diffuse alveolar damage.[66] There are many factors that can cause postoperative ALI,

such as interstitial lung disease, excessive fluid administration, and intraoperative transfusion.[67]

Surgical trauma to the operative lung from mechanical handling and reperfusion injury likely accounts for some lung injury noted after thoracic surgery. Less well recognized, however, are the injurious effects of OLV to the contralateral lung. In fact, OLV-associated ALI in the nonoperative lung is more common and can affect healthy lungs even after brief periods of OLV.[68] In a meta-analysis, the incidence of postoperative ALI was found to be 4.3%, and associated mortality was 26.5%.[69] Contributing factors included intraoperative ventilation strategies characterized by high inspiratory TV defined as greater than 10 mL/kg predicted body weight, and high peak inspiratory pressures defined as greater than 28 cm H_2O, both of which lead to abnormal stretching of the fibroelastic architecture of the lung and produce an inflammatory response.[70–72]

An intraoperative ventilation strategy aimed at maintaining adequate gas exchange while protecting the lungs from inflammation can improve postoperative outcomes. The traditional approach of high TV respirations (10–12 mL/kg) to prevent atelectasis, shunting, and oxygen desaturation during OLV has proven to be harmful.[73,74] TV of 6 mL/kg is an acceptable two–lung ventilation strategy. Halving TV to 3 mL/kg during OLV may result in unacceptably low TV and dead space ventilation. An approach that includes low TV (4–6 mL/kg) and high PEEP while achieving mean airway pressures less than 25 cm H_2O is proven to reduce volutrauma, barotrauma, and atelectrauma in patients with acute respiratory distress syndrome (ARDS).[75,76] A meta-analysis comparing low (4–6 mL/kg) versus high (8–12 mL/kg) TV strategies during OLV demonstrated preserved gas exchange, lower incidence of pulmonary infiltration, and lower incidence of ARDS in the low TV group without a significant change in postoperative pulmonary complication rate or hospital length of stay.[77] Applying this approach to OLV has been recommended,[78] although some anesthesiologists remain reluctant and continue to use strategies that prioritize reducing peak airway pressures.[79]

Avoiding high peak airway pressures (>25 cm H_2O) to achieve adequate TV is an important consideration. One way to achieve adequate TV with lower peak airway pressures is by using pressure-controlled ventilation (PCV) instead of volume-controlled ventilation (VCV).[80] A meta-analysis reported significantly higher Pao_2/Fio_2 ratio and lower peak airway pressure in the PCV group compared with the VCV group; however, no clinical difference was found in $Paco_2$, mean airway pressures, and postoperative pulmonary complications.[81] Overall, the advantages of PCV during OLV include lower peak airway pressures, lower intrapulmonary shunt, and improved oxygenation; however, how these advantages contribute to overall morbidity and mortality remains uncertain.

Excessive driving pressure, calculated as plateau pressure minus PEEP, is considered an independent risk factor for mortality in ARDS.[82] The benefit of targeting lower driving pressures during ventilation for thoracic surgery has been validated.[83] Compared with conventional ventilation strategies, targeting lower driving pressures led to fewer postoperative pulmonary complications, including lower rates of pneumonia and ARDS. Although low TV is an important component of lung protective ventilation strategies during OLV, evidence suggests that without adequate PEEP, low VT alone does not prevent postoperative pulmonary complications.[84] The optimal amount of PEEP that will prevent atelectasis and hypoxia from occurring is still debated. An individualized PEEP strategy that produces the lowest driving pressure may be favored.[83]

Technological advancements in extracorporeal lung assist systems, such as extracorporeal membrane oxygenation (ECMO), have expanded the potential for complex thoracic surgery in patients with insufficient pulmonary reserve and at significant risk of ALI.[85] ECMO has been used with good outcomes in thoracic surgery cases whereby patient-specific comorbidities or anatomic derangements confer infeasible or insufficient ventilation. It is indicated in cases of severe chest trauma warranting tracheoesophageal fistula repair or esophagectomy and in contralateral lung resection in the setting of previous pneumonectomy, lung transplantation, lung volume reduction surgery, difficult OLV, and difficult airway cases.

Right Ventricular Dysfunction

Thoracic surgery and OLV present a unique situation whereby the right ventricle (RV) is exposed to sudden changes in preload, afterload, and contractility; the summative effect can quickly escalate from insignificant morphologic changes to nonischemic RV injury, RV dysfunction, and eventual RV failure.[86] Intraoperative factors that can contribute to RV changes are numerous. V/Q mismatch and resultant hypoxemia and hypercapnia during OLV cause pulmonary vasoconstriction and substantial increases in RV afterload. Mechanical ventilation strategies that promote inflammation will negatively affect RV morphology. The mode of mechanical ventilation chosen intraoperatively can contribute. PCV has been shown to be more protective than VCV.[87] Thoracic epidural analgesia (TEA), if used for perioperative pain control, can cause loss of vasomotor tone and result in peripheral venous pooling, significantly decreasing RV preload. TEA also inhibits the native positive inotropic response of the RV to acute increases in pulmonary vascular resistance. The degree of RV dysfunction may be more severe in the setting of preexisting RV dysfunction or intraoperative factors, such as extensive thoracic surgery, bleeding, hypervolemia, or tachyarrhythmias. Several strategies exist to mitigate RV strain during OLV (**Table 4**).[86]

Vasoactive agents can be used to optimize RV function during thoracic surgery. Norepinephrine has been shown to improve RV-PA coupling, cardiac output, and RV performance in acute RV dysfunction with PA hypertension; however, high doses can increase pulmonary vascular resistance beyond systemic vascular resistance and should be avoided.[88] Vasopressin may be considered superior to norepinephrine because of endothelial nitric oxide stimulation in the pulmonary vascular

---

Table 4
Intraoperative strategies to protect right ventricular function during thoracic surgery and one-lung ventilation

Ventilation Strategies	Hemodynamic Strategies
Pressure control ventilation	Consider transesophageal echocardiography
Low TV (4–6 mL/kg)	Maintenance of sinus rhythm
Plateau pressure <25 cm H_2O	GDFT
Driving pressure <18 cm H_2O	Optimize RV preload
Avoid hypoxemia	Decrease RV afterload
Avoid hypercapnia	Increase RV contractility
	TEA
	Avoid hypothermia
	Avoid acidemia

tree at low doses (0.01-0.03 U/min), thus causing pulmonary vasodilation, but this effect is lost at higher doses, causing coronary vasoconstriction and significant reduction in RV stroke volume.[89] RV contractility can be enhanced by positive inotropes, such as epinephrine, or by inodilators, such as dobutamine, milrinone, enoximone, and levosimendan, with or without a peripheral vasoconstrictor. Lung transplantation–related RV dysfunction and pulmonary hypertension can be minimized by iNO and prostacyclin, 2 potent pulmonary vasodilators.[90]

INTRAOPERATIVE ANESTHETIC CONSIDERATIONS
Maintenance of Anesthesia

The pharmacologic choice to maintain general anesthesia has been widely debated. Inhaled anesthetics are known to inhibit HPV, whereas TIVA techniques do not. It has been theorized that TIVA would decrease V/Q mismatch and improve oxygenation, rendering TIVA the anesthetic of choice for OLV.[91] More recent data suggest that oxygenation during OLV is similar between propofol-based anesthesia and isoflurane.[92] Therefore, other factors must be considered when choosing an anesthetic. Volatile anesthetics have been shown to attenuate the inflammatory response and protect the glycocalyx of the lung parenchyma,[93–96] and do not appear to exacerbate hypoxemia.[97]

Fluid Management

A targeted fluid administration strategy for thoracic surgery is an important aspect of reducing postoperative ALI while minimizing end-organ injury.[98] Practice has changed since the deleterious effects of liberal fluid administration in pneumonectomy were first documented.[99] Today, euvolemia is the primary goal of intraoperative fluid management in lung resection and esophagectomy surgery. Attaining this goal entails navigating the balance between extreme ends of the fluid therapy spectrum to achieve an ideal lung water state.

Excessive fluid administration in lung resection can cause postoperative pulmonary edema, ARDS, reintubation, and pneumonia.[99–101] In esophagectomy, ARDS, pneumonia, prolonged intensive care unit (ICU) stays,[102] and increased morbidity[103] and mortality[104] correlate with fluid overload strategies.

Fluid restrictive strategies during major surgery are associated with a significant risk of perioperative acute kidney injury (AKI).[105] Colloid solutions that maximize the capillary oncotic load and minimize interstitial edema can inadvertently cause

AKI.[106,107] AKI in both lung resection and esophagectomy is associated with greater morbidity.[107]

Ideal fluid management strategies remain controversial. The use of dynamic hemodynamic parameters to target fluid administration, called goal-directed fluid therapy (GDFT), has been adopted by fast-track surgery experts in elective lung surgery. GDFT is now a cornerstone of most perioperative strategies to expedite patient recovery while minimizing postoperative complications.[108] GDFT strategies driven by objective data, such as pulse pressure variation and stroke volume variation, are gaining favor, although some strategies rely on the relationship between heart and lung interactions and are not as reliable in open thoracotomy.[109]

Pain Management

Multimodal pain management strategies aim to provide adequate postoperative analgesia while reducing the reliance on opioids. In addition to oral and intravenous nonopioids, regional anesthesia is commonplace. TEA is the gold standard for controlling postoperative pain and a foundation of accelerated recovery pathways in thoracic surgery.[110] In routinely used doses, TEA does not significantly affect oxygenation and might prevent the development of ALI and associated postoperative pulmonary complications.[111] Alternative regional anesthesia techniques, such as paravertebral block, erector spinae block, and serratus anterior block, can provide adequate postoperative pain relief with less systemic hypotension, but require additional specialized training and may have limited efficacy.[112]

SUMMARY

Preoperative assessment and risk-stratification of the prospective thoracic surgery patient, including the risk of developing hypoxemia during OLV, are crucial in formulating an appropriate intraoperative anesthetic plan. Hypoxemia, ALI, and right ventricular dysfunction are significant complications of OLV. Anesthesiologists should be prepared to navigate these problems and methodically choose a patient-specific management plan that mitigates perioperative morbidity. Ventilator management strategy, GDFT, and perioperative pain control are important components for optimizing postoperative recovery after thoracic surgery.

DISCLOSURE

The authors have nothing to disclose.

REFERENCES

1. McGrath B, Tennuci C, Lee G. The history of one-lung anesthesia and the double-lumen tube. J Anesth Hist 2017;3(3):76–86.

2. Falzon D, Alston RP, Coley E, et al. Lung isolation for thoracic surgery: from inception to evidence-based. J Cardiothorac Vasc Anesth 2017;31(2):678–93.

3. Zhang Y, Yan W, Fan Z, et al. Preemptive one lung ventilation enhances lung collapse during thoracoscopic surgery: a randomized controlled trial. Thorac Cancer 2019;10(6):1448–52.

4. Carlens E. A new flexible double-lumen catheter for bronchospirometry. J Thorac Surg 1949;18(5):742–6.

5. Robertshaw FL. Low resistance double-lumen endobronchial tubes. Br J Anaesth 1962;34:576–9.

6. Brodsky JB, Lemmens HJ. Left double-lumen tubes: clinical experience with 1,170 patients. J Cardiothorac Vasc Anesth 2003;17(3):289–98.

7. Brodsky JB, Macario A, Mark JB. Tracheal diameter predicts double-lumen tube size: a method for selecting left double-lumen tubes. Anesth Analg 1996;82(4):861–4.

8. Sustic A, Miletic D, Protic A, et al. Can ultrasound be useful for predicting the size of a left double-lumen bronchial tube? Tracheal width as measured by ultrasonography versus computed tomography. J Clin Anesth 2008;20(4):247–52.

9. Roldi E, Inghileri P, Dransart-Raye O, et al. Use of tracheal ultrasound combined with clinical parameters to select left double-lumen tube size: a prospective observational study. Eur J Anaesthesiol 2019;36(3):215–20.

10. Lohser J, Brodsky JB. Undersizing left double-lumen tubes. Anesth Analg 2008;107(1):342.

11. Sustic A, Protic A, Cicvaric T, et al. The addition of a brief ultrasound examination to clinical assessment increases the ability to confirm placement of double-lumen endotracheal tubes. J Clin Anesth 2010;22(4):246–9.

12. Moritz A, Irouschek A, Birkholz T, et al. The EZ-blocker for one-lung ventilation in patients undergoing thoracic surgery: clinical applications and experience in 100 cases in a routine clinical setting. J Cardiothorac Surg 2018;13(1):77.

13. Narayanaswamy M, McRae K, Slinger P, et al. Choosing a lung isolation device for thoracic surgery: a randomized trial of three bronchial blockers versus double-lumen tubes. Anesth Analg 2009;108(4):1097–101.

14. Campos JH. Lung isolation techniques for patients with difficult airway. Curr Opin Anaesthesiol 2010;23(1):12–7.

15. Knoll H, Ziegeler S, Schreiber JU, et al. Airway injuries after one-lung ventilation: a comparison between double-lumen tube and endobronchial blocker: a randomized, prospective, controlled trial. Anesthesiology 2006;105(3):471–7.

16. Honikman R, Rodriguez-Diaz CA, Cohen E. A ballooning crisis: three cases of bronchial blocker malfunction and a review. J Cardiothorac Vasc Anesth 2017;31(5):1799–804.

17. Soto RG, Oleszak SP. Resection of the Arndt bronchial blocker during stapler resection of the left lower lobe. J Cardiothorac Vasc Anesth 2006;20(1):131–2.

18. Neustein SM. Pro: bronchial blockers should be used routinely for providing one-lung ventilation. J Cardiothorac Vasc Anesth 2015;29(1):234–6.

19. Brodsky JB. Con: a bronchial blocker is not a substitute for a double-lumen endobronchial tube. J Cardiothorac Vasc Anesth 2015;29(1):237–9.

20. Shelley B, Macfie A, Kinsella J. Anesthesia for thoracic surgery: a survey of UK practice. J Cardiothorac Vasc Anesth 2011;25(6):1014–7.

21. Campos JH, Hallam EA, Ueda K. Lung isolation in the morbidly obese patient: a comparison of a left-sided double-lumen tracheal tube with the Arndt(R) wire-guided blocker. Br J Anaesth 2012;109(4):630–5.

22. Clayton-Smith A, Bennett K, Alston RP, et al. A comparison of the efficacy and adverse effects of double-lumen endobronchial tubes and bronchial blockers in thoracic surgery: a systematic review and meta-analysis of randomized controlled trials. J Cardiothorac Vasc Anesth 2015;29(4):955–66.

23. Campos JH, Feider A. Hypoxia during one-lung ventilation-a review and update. J Cardiothorac Vasc Anesth 2018;32(5):2330–8.

24. Wang M, Gong Q, Wei W. Estimation of shunt fraction by transesophageal echocardiography during one-lung ventilation. J Clin Monit Comput 2015;29(2):307–11.

25. Lumb AB, Slinger P. Hypoxic pulmonary vasoconstriction: physiology and anesthetic implications. Anesthesiology 2015;122(4):932–46.

26. Slinger P, Suissa S, Triolet W. Predicting arterial oxygenation during one-lung anaesthesia. Can J Anaesth 1992;39(10):1030–5.

27. Wang C, Guo M, Zhang N, et al. Association of body mass index and outcomes following lobectomy for non-small-cell lung cancer. World J Surg Oncol 2018;16(1):90.

28. Bardoczky GI, Szegedi LL, d'Hollander AA, et al. Two-lung and one-lung ventilation in patients with chronic obstructive pulmonary disease: the effects of position and F(IO)2. Anesth Analg 2000;90(1):35–41.

29. Klingstedt C, Hedenstierna G, Baehrendtz S, et al. Ventilation-perfusion relationships and atelectasis formation in the supine and lateral positions

during conventional mechanical and differential ventilation. Acta Anaesthesiol Scand 1990;34(6): 421–9.

30. Schwarzkopf K, Schreiber T, Bauer R, et al. The effects of increasing concentrations of isoflurane and desflurane on pulmonary perfusion and systemic oxygenation during one-lung ventilation in pigs. Anesth Analg 2001;93(6):1434–8 [table of contents].

31. Bickler PE, Feiner JR, Lipnick MS, et al. Effects of acute, profound hypoxia on healthy humans: implications for safety of tests evaluating pulse oximetry or tissue oximetry performance. Anesth Analg 2017;124(1):146–53.

32. Grocott MP, Martin DS, Levett DZ, et al. Arterial blood gases and oxygen content in climbers on Mount Everest. N Engl J Med 2009;360(2):140–9.

33. Jouett NP, Watenpaugh DE, Dunlap ME, et al. Interactive effects of hypoxia, hypercapnia and lung volume on sympathetic nerve activity in humans. Exp Physiol 2015;100(9):1018–29.

34. Meyhoff CS, Staehr AK, Rasmussen LS. Rational use of oxygen in medical disease and anesthesia. Curr Opin Anaesthesiol 2012;25(3):363–70.

35. Unzueta C, Tusman G, Suarez-Sipmann F, et al. Alveolar recruitment improves ventilation during thoracic surgery: a randomized controlled trial. Br J Anaesth 2012;108(3):517–24.

36. Park SH, Jeon YT, Hwang JW, et al. A preemptive alveolar recruitment strategy before one-lung ventilation improves arterial oxygenation in patients undergoing thoracic surgery: a prospective randomised study. Eur J Anaesthesiol 2011;28(4): 298–302.

37. Kim N, Lee SH, Choi KW, et al. Effects of positive end-expiratory pressure on pulmonary oxygenation and biventricular function during one-lung ventilation: a randomized crossover study. J Clin Med 2019;8(5) [pii:E740].

38. Cinnella G, Grasso S, Natale C, et al. Physiological effects of a lung-recruiting strategy applied during one-lung ventilation. Acta Anaesthesiol Scand 2008;52(6):766–75.

39. Tusman G, Bohm SH, Sipmann FS, et al. Lung recruitment improves the efficiency of ventilation and gas exchange during one-lung ventilation anesthesia. Anesth Analg 2004;98(6):1604–9 [table of contents].

40. Slinger PD, Kruger M, McRae K, et al. Relation of the static compliance curve and positive end-expiratory pressure to oxygenation during one-lung ventilation. Anesthesiology 2001;95(5): 1096–102.

41. Ferrando C, Mugarra A, Gutierrez A, et al. Setting individualized positive end-expiratory pressure level with a positive end-expiratory pressure decrement trial after a recruitment maneuver improves oxygenation and lung mechanics during one-lung ventilation. Anesth Analg 2014;118(3):657–65.

42. Carraminana A, Ferrando C, Unzueta MC, et al. Rationale and study design for an Individualized Perioperative Open Lung Ventilatory Strategy in Patients on One-Lung Ventilation (iPROVE-OLV). J Cardiothorac Vasc Anesth 2019;33(9): 2492–502.

43. Kiss T, Wittenstein J, Becker C, et al. Protective ventilation with high versus low positive end-expiratory pressure during one-lung ventilation for thoracic surgery (PROTHOR): study protocol for a randomized controlled trial. Trials 2019;20(1):213.

44. El Tahan MR, El Ghoneimy Y, Regal M, et al. Effects of nondependent lung ventilation with continuous positive-pressure ventilation and high-frequency positive-pressure ventilation on right ventricular function during one-lung ventilation. Semin Cardiothorac Vasc Anesth 2010;14(4):291–300.

45. Dikmen Y, Aykac B, Erolcay H. Unilateral high frequency jet ventilation during one-lung ventilation. Eur J Anaesthesiol 1997;14(3):239–43.

46. Kremer R, Aboud W, Haberfeld O, et al. Differential lung ventilation for increased oxygenation during one lung ventilation for video assisted lung surgery. J Cardiothorac Surg 2019;14(1):89.

47. Modolo NS, Modolo MP, Marton MA, et al. Intravenous versus inhalation anaesthesia for one-lung ventilation. Cochrane Database Syst Rev 2013;(7):CD006313.

48. Fradj K, Samain E, Delefosse D, et al. Placebo-controlled study of inhaled nitric oxide to treat hypoxaemia during one-lung ventilation. Br J Anaesth 1999;82(2):208–12.

49. Dalibon N, Moutafis M, Liu N, et al. Treatment of hypoxemia during one-lung ventilation using intravenous almitrine. Anesth Analg 2004;98(3):590–4 [table of contents].

50. Silva-Costa-Gomes T, Gallart L, Valles J, et al. Low- vs high-dose almitrine combined with nitric oxide to prevent hypoxia during open-chest one-lung ventilation. Br J Anaesth 2005;95(3):410–6.

51. Bermejo S, Gallart L, Silva-Costa-Gomes T, et al. Almitrine fails to improve oxygenation during one-lung ventilation with sevoflurane anesthesia. J Cardiothorac Vasc Anesth 2014;28(4):919–24.

52. Schwarzkopf K, Klein U, Schreiber T, et al. Oxygenation during one-lung ventilation: the effects of inhaled nitric oxide and increasing levels of inspired fraction of oxygen. Anesth Analg 2001; 92(4):842–7.

53. Rocca GD, Passariello M, Coccia C, et al. Inhaled nitric oxide administration during one-lung ventilation in patients undergoing thoracic surgery. J Cardiothorac Vasc Anesth 2001;15(2):218–23.

54. Choi H, Jeon J, Huh J, et al. The effects of iloprost on oxygenation during one-lung ventilation for lung

surgery: a randomized controlled trial. J Clin Med 2019;8(7) [pii:E982].

55. Lee SH, Kim N, Lee CY, et al. Effects of dexmedetomidine on oxygenation and lung mechanics in patients with moderate chronic obstructive pulmonary disease undergoing lung cancer surgery: a randomised double-blinded trial. Eur J Anaesthesiol 2016;33(4):275–82.

56. Huang SQ, Zhang J, Zhang XX, et al. Can dexmedetomidine improve arterial oxygenation and intrapulmonary shunt during one-lung ventilation in adults undergoing thoracic surgery? A meta-analysis of randomized, placebo-controlled trials. Chin Med J (Engl) 2017;130(14):1707–14.

57. Scheeren TWL, Belda FJ, Perel A. The oxygen reserve index (ORI): a new tool to monitor oxygen therapy. J Clin Monit Comput 2018;32(3): 379–89.

58. Alday E, Nieves JM, Planas A. Oxygen reserve index predicts hypoxemia during one-lung ventilation: an observational diagnostic study. J Cardiothorac Vasc Anesth 2020;34(2):417–22.

59. Koishi W, Kumagai M, Ogawa S, et al. Monitoring the oxygen reserve index can contribute to the early detection of deterioration in blood oxygenation during one-lung ventilation. Minerva Anestesiol 2018;84(9):1063–9.

60. Saugel B, Belda FJ. The oxygen reserve index in anesthesiology: a superfluous toy or a tool to individualize oxygen therapy? Minerva Anestesiol 2018;84(9):1010–2.

61. Li XM, Li F, Liu ZK, et al. Investigation of one-lung ventilation postoperative cognitive dysfunction and regional cerebral oxygen saturation relations. J Zhejiang Univ Sci B 2015;16(12):1042–8.

62. Suehiro K, Okutai R. Cerebral desaturation during single-lung ventilation is negatively correlated with preoperative respiratory functions. J Cardiothorac Vasc Anesth 2011;25(1):127–30.

63. Kazan R, Bracco D, Hemmerling TM. Reduced cerebral oxygen saturation measured by absolute cerebral oximetry during thoracic surgery correlates with postoperative complications. Br J Anaesth 2009;103(6):811–6.

64. Brinkman R, Amadeo RJ, Funk DJ, et al. Cerebral oxygen desaturation during one-lung ventilation: correlation with hemodynamic variables. Can J Anaesth 2013;60(7):660–6.

65. Tang L, Kazan R, Taddei R, et al. Reduced cerebral oxygen saturation during thoracic surgery predicts early postoperative cognitive dysfunction. Br J Anaesth 2012;108(4):623–9.

66. Katzenstein AA, Askin FB. Surgical pathology of non-neoplastic lung disease. Major Probl Pathol 1982;13:1–430.

67. Kim HJ, Cha SI, Kim CH, et al. Risk factors of postoperative acute lung injury following lobectomy for nonsmall cell lung cancer. Medicine (Baltimore) 2019;98(13):e15078.

68. Padley SP, Jordan SJ, Goldstraw P, et al. Asymmetric ARDS following pulmonary resection: CT findings initial observations. Radiology 2002; 223(2):468–73.

69. Slutsky AS, Ranieri VM. Ventilator-induced lung injury. N Engl J Med 2014;370(10):980.

70. Jordan S, Mitchell JA, Quinlan GJ, et al. The pathogenesis of lung injury following pulmonary resection. Eur Respir J 2000;15(4):790–9.

71. Schilling T, Kozian A, Huth C, et al. The pulmonary immune effects of mechanical ventilation in patients undergoing thoracic surgery. Anesth Analg 2005;101(4):957–65 [table of contents].

72. Kozian A, Schilling T, Rocken C, et al. Increased alveolar damage after mechanical ventilation in a porcine model of thoracic surgery. J Cardiothorac Vasc Anesth 2010;24(4):617–23.

73. Slinger PD. Do low tidal volumes decrease lung injury during one-lung ventilation? J Cardiothorac Vasc Anesth 2017;31(5):1774–5.

74. Gama de Abreu M, Heintz M, Heller A, et al. One-lung ventilation with high tidal volumes and zero positive end-expiratory pressure is injurious in the isolated rabbit lung model. Anesth Analg 2003; 96(1):220–8 [table of contents].

75. Serpa Neto A, Cardoso SO, Manetta JA, et al. Association between use of lung-protective ventilation with lower tidal volumes and clinical outcomes among patients without acute respiratory distress syndrome: a meta-analysis. JAMA 2012;308(16): 1651–9.

76. Acute Respiratory Distress Syndrome Network, Brower RG, Matthay MA, Morris A, et al. Ventilation with lower tidal volumes as compared with traditional tidal volumes for acute lung injury and the acute respiratory distress syndrome. N Engl J Med 2000;342(18):1301–8.

77. El Tahan MR, Pasin L, Marczin N, et al. Impact of low tidal volumes during one-lung ventilation. A meta-analysis of randomized controlled trials. J Cardiothorac Vasc Anesth 2017;31(5):1767–73.

78. Serpa Neto A, Hemmes SN, Barbas CS, et al. Protective versus conventional ventilation for surgery: a systematic review and individual patient data meta-analysis. Anesthesiology 2015;123(1):66–78.

79. Kidane B, Choi S, Fortin D, et al. Use of lung-protective strategies during one-lung ventilation surgery: a multi-institutional survey. Ann Transl Med 2018;6(13):269.

80. Yang M, Ahn HJ, Kim K, et al. Does a protective ventilation strategy reduce the risk of pulmonary complications after lung cancer surgery?: a randomized controlled trial. Chest 2011;139(3):530–7.

81. Kim KN, Kim DW, Jeong MA, et al. Comparison of pressure-controlled ventilation with volume-

controlled ventilation during one-lung ventilation: a systematic review and meta-analysis. BMC Anesthesiol 2016;16(1):72.

82. Amato MB, Meade MO, Slutsky AS, et al. Driving pressure and survival in the acute respiratory distress syndrome. N Engl J Med 2015;372(8): 747–55.

83. Park M, Ahn HJ, Kim JA, et al. Driving pressure during thoracic surgery: a randomized clinical trial. Anesthesiology 2019;130(3):385–93.

84. Blank RS, Colquhoun DA, Durieux ME, et al. Management of one-lung ventilation: impact of tidal volume on complications after thoracic surgery. Anesthesiology 2016;124(6):1286–95.

85. McRae K, de Perrot M. Principles and indications of extracorporeal life support in general thoracic surgery. J Thorac Dis 2018;10(Suppl 8):S931–46.

86. Rana M, Yusuff H, Zochios V. The right ventricle during selective lung ventilation for thoracic surgery. J Cardiothorac Vasc Anesth 2019;33(7): 2007–16.

87. Al Shehri AM, El-Tahan MR, Al Metwally R, et al. Right ventricular function during one-lung ventilation: effects of pressure-controlled and volume-controlled ventilation. J Cardiothorac Vasc Anesth 2014;28(4):880–4.

88. Hirsch LJ, Rooney MW, Wat SS, et al. Norepinephrine and phenylephrine effects on right ventricular function in experimental canine pulmonary embolism. Chest 1991;100(3):796–801.

89. Leather HA, Segers P, Berends N, et al. Effects of vasopressin on right ventricular function in an experimental model of acute pulmonary hypertension. Crit Care Med 2002;30(11):2548–52.

90. Ardehali A, Laks H, Levine M, et al. A prospective trial of inhaled nitric oxide in clinical lung transplantation. Transplantation 2001;72(1):112–5.

91. Schwarzkopf K, Schreiber T, Preussler NP, et al. Lung perfusion, shunt fraction, and oxygenation during one-lung ventilation in pigs: the effects of desflurane, isoflurane, and propofol. J Cardiothorac Vasc Anesth 2003;17(1):73–5.

92. Sheybani S, Attar AS, Golshan S, et al. Effect of propofol and isoflurane on gas exchange parameters following one-lung ventilation in thoracic surgery: a double-blinded randomized controlled clinical trial. Electron Physician 2018;10(2): 6346–53.

93. Schilling T, Kozian A, Senturk M, et al. Effects of volatile and intravenous anesthesia on the alveolar and systemic inflammatory response in thoracic surgical patients. Anesthesiology 2011;115(1): 65–74.

94. De Conno E, Steurer MP, Wittlinger M, et al. Anesthetic-induced improvement of the inflammatory response to one-lung ventilation. Anesthesiology 2009;110(6):1316–26.

95. Sun B, Wang J, Bo L, et al. Effects of volatile vs. propofol-based intravenous anesthetics on the alveolar inflammatory responses to one-lung ventilation: a meta-analysis of randomized controlled trials. J Anesth 2015;29(4):570–9.

96. Chappell D, Heindl B, Jacob M, et al. Sevoflurane reduces leukocyte and platelet adhesion after ischemia-reperfusion by protecting the endothelial glycocalyx. Anesthesiology 2011;115(3):483–91.

97. Ng A, Swanevelder J. Hypoxaemia associated with one-lung anaesthesia: new discoveries in ventilation and perfusion. Br J Anaesth 2011;106(6): 761–3.

98. Ashes CSP. Volume management and resuscitation in thoracic surgery. Curr Anesthesiol Rep 2014;4: 386–96.

99. Zeldin RA, Normandin D, Landtwing D, et al. Postpneumonectomy pulmonary edema. J Thorac Cardiovasc Surg 1984;87(3):359–65.

100. Turnage WS, Lunn JJ. Postpneumonectomy pulmonary edema. A retrospective analysis of associated variables. Chest 1993;103(6):1646–50.

101. Arslantas MK, Kara HV, Tuncer BB, et al. Effect of the amount of intraoperative fluid administration on postoperative pulmonary complications following anatomic lung resections. J Thorac Cardiovasc Surg 2015;149(1):314–20, 321.e1.

102. Casado D, Lopez F, Marti R. Perioperative fluid management and major respiratory complications in patients undergoing esophagectomy. Dis Esophagus 2010;23(7):523–8.

103. Eng OS, Arlow RL, Moore D, et al. Fluid administration and morbidity in transhiatal esophagectomy. J Surg Res 2016;200(1):91–7.

104. Glatz T, Kulemann B, Marjanovic G, et al. Postoperative fluid overload is a risk factor for adverse surgical outcome in patients undergoing esophagectomy for esophageal cancer: a retrospective study in 335 patients. BMC Surg 2017; 17(1):6.

105. Myles PS, Bellomo R, Corcoran T, et al. Restrictive versus liberal fluid therapy for major abdominal surgery. N Engl J Med 2018;378(24):2263–74.

106. Jo JY, Kim WJ, Choi DK, et al. Effect of restrictive fluid therapy with hydroxyethyl starch during esophagectomy on postoperative outcomes: a retrospective cohort study. BMC Surg 2019; 19(1):15.

107. Ahn HJ, Kim JA, Lee AR, et al. The risk of acute kidney injury from fluid restriction and hydroxyethyl starch in thoracic surgery. Anesth Analg 2016; 122(1):186–93.

108. Batchelor TJP, Rasburn NJ, Abdelnour-Berchtold E, et al. Guidelines for enhanced recovery after lung surgery: recommendations of the Enhanced Recovery After Surgery (ERAS(R)) Society and the European Society of Thoracic Surgeons

(ESTS). Eur J Cardiothorac Surg 2019;55(1): 91–115.

109. Lee JH, Jeon Y, Bahk JH, et al. Pulse pressure variation as a predictor of fluid responsiveness during one-lung ventilation for lung surgery using thoracotomy: randomised controlled study. Eur J Anaesthesiol 2011;28(1):39–44.

110. Senturk M, Ozcan PE, Talu GK, et al. The effects of three different analgesia techniques on long-term postthoracotomy pain. Anesth Analg 2002;94(1): 11–5 [table of contents].

111. Ozcan PE, Senturk M, Sungur Ulke Z, et al. Effects of thoracic epidural anaesthesia on pulmonary venous admixture and oxygenation during one-lung ventilation. Acta Anaesthesiol Scand 2007; 51(8):1117–22.

112. Elmore B, Nguyen V, Blank R, et al. Pain management following thoracic surgery. Thorac Surg Clin 2015;25(4):393–409.

Intraoperative Anesthetic and Surgical Concerns for Robotic Thoracic Surgery

Travis C. Geraci, MD[a],*, Prabhu Sasankan, BS[b], Brent Luria, MD[c],
Robert J. Cerfolio, MD, MBA[a]

KEYWORDS

- Robotic surgery • Anesthesia • Complications • Conversion • Technique • Intraoperative

KEY POINTS

- Anesthetic considerations for thoracic surgery are evolving concomitant with the shift from open to minimally invasive surgery, including the use of robotic systems.
- Successful robotic surgery begins with optimal patient positioning and port placement, which are particular to the planned operating and target anatomy.
- Robotic pulmonary resection is aided by new technologies, including the use of contrast agents to localize pulmonary nodules and define the intersegmental planes.
- Catastrophic events during robotic thoracic surgery are uncommon, but surgeons must be prepared to address them effectively, which may include conversion to open thoracotomy.

INTRODUCTION

A robotic approach has been applied to nearly all procedures in the chest, including surgery of the lung, esophagus, and mediastinum, with outstanding short-term outcomes. With this shift in technology, the intraoperative anesthetic and surgical concerns have equally changed. With less surgical stress during minimally invasive surgery, anesthetic monitoring and approaches to pain control have become more conservative. From a surgical perspective, greater visualization of structures on the robotic system has come with the loss of tactile feedback, creating new challenges. In this review, we discuss the intraoperative anesthetic and surgical concerns as they pertain to pulmonary, esophageal, and mediastinal thoracic robotic operations.

ANESTHETIC MANAGEMENT IN ROBOTIC THORACIC SURGERY

The evolving shift away from open thoracotomy to minimally invasive techniques in thoracic surgery has changed the fundamental anesthetic concerns for these operations. Anesthetic management for robotic lung surgery, is similar to the management of patients undergoing video-assisted thoracoscopic surgery (VATS), typically with general anesthetic technique and controlled, one-lung ventilation.

One-Lung Ventilation

During robotic pulmonary resection, selective ventilation of the nonoperative lung with deflation of the operative lung, or one-lung ventilation, provides a surgical space in the closed thoracic

Acknowledgments/Funding Statement: Dr T.C. Geraci, Mr P. Sasankan, and Dr B. Luria have no disclosures. Dr R. J. Cerfolio discloses past relationships with AstraZeneca, Bard Davol, Bovie Medical Corporation, C-SATS, ConMed, Covidien/Medtronic, Ethicon, Fruit Street Health, Google/Verb Surgical, Intuitive Surgical, KCI/Acelity, Myriad Genetics, Neomend, Pinnacle Biologics, ROLO-7, Tego, and TransEnterix.
[a] Department of Cardiothoracic Surgery, New York University Langone Health, New York, NY, USA; [b] New York University School of Medicine, NYU Langone Health, 550 1st Avenue, 15th Floor, New York, NY 10016, USA; [c] Department of Anesthesiology, New York University Langone Health, 550 1st Avenue, 15th Floor, New York, NY 10016, USA
* Corresponding author. Department of Cardiothoracic Surgery, New York University Langone Health, 550 1st Avenue, 15th Floor, New York, NY 10016.
E-mail address: travis.geraci@nyulangone.org

Thorac Surg Clin 30 (2020) 293–304
https://doi.org/10.1016/j.thorsurg.2020.04.006
1547-4127/20/© 2020 Elsevier Inc. All rights reserved.

cavity. One-lung ventilation can be attained through several different methods, including placement of a bronchial blocker, although use of a double lumen tube is the most effective and efficient and, therefore, most commonly used method.

Ventilation strategies for robotic lung surgery mirror those for any other thoracic surgery in which one-lung ventilation is used. Preoxygenation with 100% inspired oxygen before lung isolation theoretically decreases the nitrogen concentration of the lungs, facilitating rapid lung deflation via expedient absorption of oxygen. Protective single lung ventilation strategies should be used to prevent barotrauma to the ventilated lung and to avoid postoperative pulmonary dysfunction. Different methods exist to determine the optimal tidal volume and positive end-expiratory pressure to be delivered. Titration of the fraction of inspired oxygen and small increments of positive end-expiratory pressure can be applied to prevent and/or treat intraoperative hypoxia.

Operative visualization is improved with the instillation of carbon dioxide into the operative chest. The pressurized pneumothorax achieves a more rapid and permanent deflation of the lungs when compared with passive deflation. Further, a pressured chest deflects the diaphragm into the abdomen created a wider surgical field. Venous return to the heart may be impeded with high intrathoracic pressure, typically occurring only when the pressure exceeds 5 mm Hg. For this reason, a patient's blood pressure should always be check immediately after the initiation of insufflation. When hypotension develops, the operation is held and insufflation pressure is decreased until hemodynamics have normalized. Rare occurrences of carbon dioxide embolism have been reported when the system is erroneously placed in the lung parenchyma.[1] Severe subcutaneous emphysema can result when placed in the extrathoracic tissues.

Monitoring and Access

Patient monitoring for robotic lung surgery incorporates the standard American Society of Anesthesiologists monitors: electrocardiogram, pulse oximetry, capnography, and noninvasive blood pressure cuff.

We do not use arterial lines routinely, but place them selectively in patients with severe cardiac morbidity or for anticipated operative complexity. Traditionally, arterial line monitoring was used in the vast majority of thoracic surgical procedures, both owing to the risk of intraoperative blood loss and to monitor blood gasses during 1 lung ventilation. As anesthesiologists have become more experienced with minimally invasive thoracic surgery, the imperative to reflexively place arterial cannulas for these procedures has largely abated. For more complicated cases, including bilobectomy, esophagectomy, reoperative cases, and more invasive surgical procedures with higher potential for blood loss and hemodynamic compromise, it is prudent to place an arterial cannula for beat-to-beat monitoring of the blood pressure and for the ability to draw arterial blood samples for intraoperative analysis.

A single, medium-sized intravenous line is often sufficient for the majority of cases. Venous access with multiple large-bore intravenous lines, or even a central line, is generally unnecessary, but may be considered for difficult operations, which may complicate intraoperative hemodynamic status, such as patients with sepsis from empyema or esophageal preformation. One caveat to the emphasis on minimizing the placement of lines is the challenge of direct physical access to the patient associated with positioning for robotic surgery. Although the lateral positioning is similar to that of VATS and open thoracotomy, the positioning of the surgical robot often limits access by the anesthesiologist to the patient's arm and face. This can present a challenge if the need for placement of additional venous access or an arterial catheter arises during the course of the surgery. The Xi system is the current edition of the da Vinci robot and provides greater versatility and functionality. The Xi system allows for docking of the robot to the side of the operating table, whereas the Si system requires placement of the robotic cart at the patient's head. With the greater maneuverability of the Xi, patient access for the anesthesiologist is significantly enhanced.

The incidence of postoperative urinary retention in the literature varies from 5% to 70% and is complicated by the lack of consistent definitions, variance in surgical procedures and populations, and differences in the administration of anesthetic agents.[2] Established risk factors include older age, male sex, type of perioperative and intraoperative anesthetics and analgesics administered, and the type and duration of surgery. The placement of a urinary catheter is infrequently required, except in patients at high risk for postoperative urinary retention (patients with benign prostatic hyperplasia) or when the operation is expected to last more than 3 hours.

Pain Management

In the era of enhanced recovery for surgery, the importance of controlling postoperative pain is critical to decreasing postoperative morbidity, decreasing length of hospital stay, and improving patient satisfaction. Enhanced recovery protocols assist the entire perioperative team in planning ahead and minimizing both the magnitude and duration of patients' postoperative pain. Crucial to that goal is a well-designed perioperative analgesic protocol. Our preferred preemptive regimen includes acetaminophen and gabapentin, taken orally before surgery. Multimodal analgesia allows for the synergistic combination of drugs with varying mechanisms of action and helps to minimize side effects by requiring lower doses of the individual analgesic agents. Specifically, the combination of preoperative oral medications and intraoperative nerve blockade allows for the minimization of opioid administration, both in the operating room and in the immediate postoperative period. This strategy minimizes opioid-related side effects and facilitates early ambulation and hospital discharge.

The need for invasive pain management procedures, such as thoracic epidural catheter placement or paravertebral blocks, has decreased with smaller incisions and lower postoperative pain experienced by patients after minimally invasive thoracic surgery. Regional anesthetic techniques help to attenuate endocrine and metabolic responses to the stress of surgery, limiting stress-induced organ dysfunction and pain postoperatively.[3] We routinely perform a subpleural paravertebral intercostal block with bupivacaine hydrochloride (Marcaine). Performance of intercostal nerve blockade is done under direct visualization with the robotic camera. Additionally, we instill local anesthetic at each port site in the subcutaneous tissue as a field block. The optimal admixture of local anesthetic for pleural and subcutaneous blockade is controversial. Presently, we do not feel the need for additives above a long-acting local anesthetic, such as epinephrine, steroids, or liposomal bupivacaine (Exparel). Retrospective studies have shown conflicting data regarding liposomal bupivacaine in patients undergoing thoracotomy or thoracoscopy.[4,5] In a randomized controlled trial, liposomal bupivacaine marginally decreased postoperative pain and failed to provide an opioid-sparing benefit to patients after sternotomy.[6]

Fluid Management

Administration of large volumes of fluid during thoracic surgery is a contributory, if not causative, factor in the development of postoperative complications. A number of studies have shown that fluid administration of more than 2 L is associated with

pulmonary edema and acute lung injury.[7] Our goal is to limit fluid volume to less than 1 L for every thoracic surgery case. Fluid requirements or more than 1 L should prompt a discussion between the anesthesiologist and surgeon regarding the operative plan and hemodynamic status.

Intraoperative Communication

Strong communication between members of the operative team is imperative for safe and efficient robotic surgery. During robotic surgery, the surgeon is positioned on the surgeon console, which is typically distant from the patient and anesthesiologist. Despite amplified microphones and operative speakers, communication between members of the team is inherently less intimate and direct than open surgery at the surgical table. Communication must be clear and concise. To help encourage communication, we do not pin up the surgical drapes at the patient's head, but allow the sterile field to fall, permitting a clear line of vision between all members of the team. Talkback techniques to confirm understanding is an effective tool for avoiding errors and miscues. Ambient noise is amplified in the surgeon console and can be distracting. We advise a quiet operating room to maximize team communication, particularly during critical parts of the case. Maintaining a relatively small group of anesthesiologists, physician assistants, circulating nurses, and scrub techs, all of whom are very familiar with the unique elements of robotic thoracic surgery, helps to foster a collaborative atmosphere and to facilitate communication between the members of the team.

PATIENT AND PORT POSITIONING

Safe and efficient patient position is essential for successful robotic thoracic surgery. Despite the operation performed, care is taken to adequately pad the patient's arms and legs, using foam positioners, pillows, and blankets to buffer any zone where the patient's body will be pressed. We attempt to limit the number of support systems used, avoiding the use of beanbags, axillary rolls, or arm boards. The patient is secured to the operating table at the hip, shoulders, upper extremities, and at the legs.

Robotic instruments are inserted via trocars, which are placed between the ribs through intercostal incisions. The arms incorporate remote center technology that anchors the fulcrum of the robotic arms in space, thereby reducing stress to the ribs. Despite the relative stability of the trocars, lateral and pivoting movements of robotic instruments produce pressure on the intercostal nerves, contributing to postoperative pain and dysfunction. To limit nerve trauma, it is important that the robotic trocars are driven straight into the chest, avoiding angulation, thereby limiting pressure on the intercostal nerve. We use a zero-degree camera to continue minimizing the torque placed on the intercostal nerve at the camera port.

Successful robotic surgery also depends on a skilled bedside assistant. Given the coordination required between surgeon, assistant, and the robotic system, a dedicated assistant with familiarity with the conduct of the operation provides continuity and improves efficiency.

The lateral decubitus position is used for robotic pulmonary resection and thoracic mobilization and reconstruction during esophagectomy. A mild degree of flexion is used to increase the space between the intercostal spaces and to displace the hip from the chest, allowing greater range of motion at the assistant port.

Pulmonary Resections

Port sites are initially mapped on the patient to guide placement. The ports are placed in the eighth intercostal space, above the ninth rib: robotic arm 3 (8-mm port) is placed 4 cm from the lateral aspect of the spinous process of the vertebral body, robotic arm 2 (8 mm) is 8 cm medial to robotic arm 3, the camera port is 8 cm medial to robotic arm 2, and robotic arm 1 (12 mm) is placed approximately 8 cm medial to the camera port, avoiding the rectus muscles, just above the diaphragm (**Fig. 1**). The assistant port is triangulated behind the most anterior robotic port and the camera port. Typically, robotic arm 1 is the "right hand," which controls a bipolar forceps. Robotic arm 2 is the "left hand" and typically controls a grasper, such as a Cadiere forceps. Robotic arm 4 typically controls a tips-up grasper, which is used for retraction and blunt dissection.

Esophagectomy

During the thoracic phase for robotic esophagectomy, the patient is placed in the left lateral decubitus position with the right chest up and tilted forward to allow the lung to fall away from the posterior mediastinum (**Fig. 2**). The port for the right robotic arm is marked at the inferior aspect of the right axilla, just below the hairline, medial to the anterior aspect of the scapula. The arm serves as the surgeon's right hand, commonly used to control a long bipolar grasper or vessel sealer. The robotic camera port is placed 8 to 10 cm inferiorly to the right robotic arm in the same anatomic plane. The left robotic arm port is placed 8 to 10 cm inferiorly to the camera port, in the same

anatomic plane. The left hand typically controls a Cadiere forceps. An additional left-sided instrument port, which is primarily used for retraction, is placed at the posterior axillary line, just above the diaphragm.

Mediastinal Resections

Robotic mediastinal surgery can be approached from the left chest, right chest, or bilaterally. Each access strategy has its own particular advantages and disadvantages. Ultimately, the approach depends on the anatomy of the lesion, most commonly its predominant sidedness, or involvement of critical sided structures such as the phrenic nerve. A supine position, modified with the patient's ipsilateral side bumped at an approximate 30° angle, is safe and effective for robotic mediastinal surgery (**Fig. 3**). The ipsilateral arm is allowed to lay beneath the operating table on a slim arm board, exposing the operative chest. The contralateral arm is tucked to allow space for the robotic system, which is driven perpendicular to the patient from the opposite side.

Given the limited space in the anterior mediastinum, safe port positioning is necessary to avoid

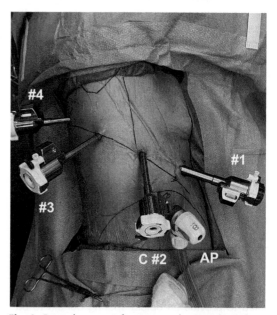

Fig. 1. Port placement for 4-arm robotic right pulmonary resection. The anatomy is mapped out on the patient to guide port placement, including the scapula, posterior axillary line, ribs 8 to 12, demarcation of the ninth rib, and estimated course of the diaphragm cresting to the 10th rib. Robotic ports/arms: anterior port, robotic arm 1, "right hand" (#1), the assistant port (AP), camera port, robotic arm 2 (C #2), posterior port, robotic arm 3, "left hand" (#3), 2nd posterior port, robotic arm 4, "retraction" (#4).

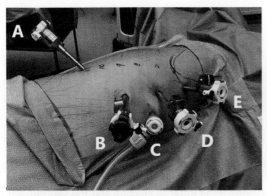

Fig. 2. Port placement for the thoracic phase of a robotic esophagectomy. (A) Additional left robotic arm, (B) left robotic arm, (C) assistant port, (D) camera port, and (E) right robotic arm.

injury, which is particularly critical in the left chest given the proximity of the heart. The camera port is placed first, approximately 1 rib space below the middle of the sternum, lateral to the pectoralis major and breast tissue. The most superior port is placed next, 2 to 3 rib spaces above the camera at the same approximate level. This port must be placed below the innominate vein to have access to the superior anterior mediastinum. The third port is on a more medial plane then the prior ports, approximately 2 to 3 cm below the breast. A 5- or 8-mm access port is triangulated between middle and inferior port. The access port incision can be extended to the inferior port to allow the removal of large specimens.

ROBOTIC PULMONARY RESECTION

The use of robotic surgical systems has accelerated over the last decade as increasing data report excellent short-term outcomes for a number of

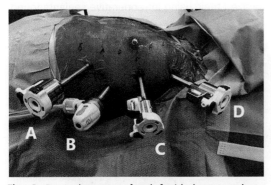

Fig. 3. Port placement for left-sided approach to resection of an anterior mediastinal mass. (A) Inferior port, more medial to the plane of the camera and superior port, (B) 8-mm assistant port, (C) camera port, and (D) superior port.

operations, including pulmonary lobectomy. Robotic pulmonary lobectomy for non-small cell lung cancer has been shown to be safe and effective, with superior short-term postoperative outcomes when compared with lobectomy via open thoracotomy, and relative parity of outcomes when compared with VATS.[8] Long-term outcomes after robotic lobectomy are promising, with a 5-year stage-specific survival of 83% for stage IA non-small cell lung cancer, 77% for stage IB, 68% for stage IIA, 70% for IIB, 62% IIIA, and 31% for IIIB (seventh edition, lung cancer staging) with an incidence of 3% for local recurrence in the ipsilateral operated chest.[9]

Localization of Pulmonary Nodules

Small pulmonary nodules (<2 cm), or those with a subsolid or ground glass composition, are often difficult to identify during minimally invasive pulmonary resection. With a lack of haptic feedback and reliance on visual distortion of the parenchyma, intraoperative localization of these nodules is even more difficult on the robotic system. When performing lobectomy, a preoperative computed tomography scan may be enough to determine nodule location; however, during segmentectomy, nodules may be more difficult to locate and may exist between adjacent segments.

There are many methods for intraoperative nodule localization, including radiographically placed wires, coils, or markers, and the use of injected contrast agents. The use of electromagnetic navigational bronchoscopy using near-infrared fluorescence with indocyanine green contrast (ICG) has emerged as an accurate and efficient method for localizing pulmonary nodules (Fig. 4). In a series of patients who underwent planned robotic segmentectomy, we selected 93 for electromagnetic navigational bronchoscopy localization with ICG owing to small nodule size and/or challenging anatomic location (between segments or deep to the visceral pleural surface). Of the 93 patients undergoing electromagnetic navigational bronchoscopy, we successfully identified the pulmonary nodule in 80 patients (86%).[10]

Segmentectomy

Prospective nonrandomized data have shown comparable long-term survival in patients undergoing sublobar resection versus lobectomy with nodules less than 2 cm without nodal metastasis.[11] Two prospective, randomized clinical trials—the Cancer and Leukemia Group B Trial 140503 and the Japan Clinical Oncology Group 0802/WJOG 4607L and JCOG 1211 Trial—are currently being conducted to help address the

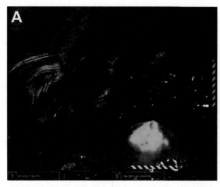 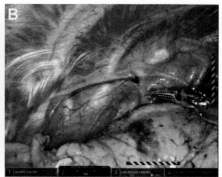

Fig. 4. Localization of a pulmonary nodule in the left upper lobe using infrared imaging and ICG contrast. (*A*) Firefly infrared camera. (*B*) Robotic camera.

oncologic outcomes after sublobar resection versus lobectomy in patients with early stage non-small cell lung cancer.[12]

To help accurately define the intersegmental plane during segmentectomy, thereby assuring the correct division of the anatomic segment and maintaining an appropriate tumor margin, ICG contrast can be administered intravenously after ligation of the corresponding pulmonary artery. A clear delineation of the tissue is illuminated with infrared imaging (**Fig. 5**). Further, this method avoids inflation–deflation of the lung, which obscures the operative view and may be inaccurate given the continuity of the pulmonary parenchyma with pores of Kohn.

Prevention of Air Leak

Most air leaks after pulmonary resection are alveolar–pleural fistulas, a communication between the pulmonary parenchyma distal to a segmental bronchus and the pleural space. Alveolar–pleural fistulas are very common, occurring in about one-third of patients after elective pulmonary resection. Prolonged air leaks increase

length of stay and financial costs, and delay chest tube removal increasing postoperative pain and risk of infection. Several risk factors can increase the risk of air leak, including the use of chronic steroids, emphysematous lung disease, and larger resections that leave a pleural space deficit.

During robotic pulmonary resection, it is imperative to avoid puncturing the lung during initial port placement. Despite single lung ventilation, the lung may remain adherent to the chest wall either by normal pleural apposition or from the formation of pleural adhesions secondary to prior surgery, tube thoracostomy, neoadjuvant therapy, or an inflammatory pleural process. If a puncture occurs, these defects should be repaired with an interrupted suture.

Tissue handling to avoid parenchymal tearing decreases the risk of postoperative air leak. Large areas of denuded visceral pleura or lymph node basins with dense adherence to the lung, may benefit from the application of tissue sealants such as Progel (Neomend, Irvine, CA). We use these products selectively, and only in high-risk patients after difficult dissections. A review of randomized trials using intraoperative sealants found

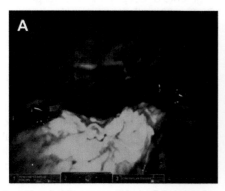 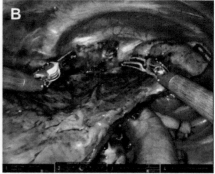

Fig. 5. Delineation of the intersegmental plane between the lingula (illuminated with ICG) and the remaining left upper lobe, during robotic left upper lobe trisegmentectomy. (*A*) Firefly infrared camera. (*B*) Robotic camera.

that these products decreased postoperative air leaks and time to removal of chest drains, however, with equivocal data regarding a decrease in the length of hospital stay.[13]

For the majority of air leaks, water seal is superior to suction and promotes earlier resolution. For large leaks, suction may be required to prevent the development of subcutaneous emphysema or hypoxia.[14] Patients with a large or persistent air leak, which we define as one that delays the patient's discharge, can be sent home with an outpatient drainage device. For these patients, the chest tube can usually be removed in the clinic approximately 1 to 2 weeks postoperatively. It is important to remove the chest tube as soon as possible, to decrease the risk of developing an empyema.[15]

ROBOTIC MEDIASTINAL SURGERY

Robotic mediastinal surgery is typically used for thymectomy in patients with an anterior mediastinal mass, most commonly for thymoma with or without myasthenia gravis. Robotic mediastinal surgery can also be used to resect soft tissue masses such as teratomas, nerve sheath tumors (schwannomas, neurofibromas), lymphomas, thyroid tumors, and parathyroid tumors or cystic structures of the hilum, esophagus or pericardium.

Robotic thymectomy involves resection of the encapsulated thymus and all surrounding perithymic and mediastinal adipose tissue. These tissues are optimally resected en bloc with the bilateral upper horns and lower poles. The borders of resection include the phrenic nerves laterally, diaphragm inferiorly, and superiorly to the cervical border of the anterior mediastinum above the innominate vein.

Anesthetic Considerations

Patients with myasthenia gravis pose unique challenges in the perioperative period. Preoperative titration of anticholinesterase blockade and steroid administration is continued to the lowest levels while maintaining baseline function and symptomatic relief. In the operating room, the neuromuscular relaxation status of patients with myasthenia gravity must be monitored closely. The stress of surgery may exacerbate preoperative muscle fatigue, which can lead to respiratory insufficiency and dependence on mechanical ventilation. At the end of the procedure, the patient is fully reversed of any residual paralysis, to minimize the risk of postoperative respiratory compromise. We typically reverse neuromuscular blockade with sugammadex (Bridion) to ensure complete return of respiratory function.

For patients undergoing resection of large masses of the anterior mediastinum, compression of the airways or heart may lead to complications. A thorough plan for maintaining the airway must be derived before the administration of muscle relaxants, because tracheobronchial obstruction may become apparent only after induction of anesthesia. If airway obstruction develops, several methods may be used to obtain an airway including rigid bronchoscopy, the use of a tracheal tube introducer (bougie), or fiberoptic intubation.

Intraoperative dissection of a large mediastinal mass may cause compression of the heart, leading to significant hypotension. It is critical to maintain communication between the surgeon and the anesthesiologist during manipulation of the mass to anticipate hemodynamic compromise and to relieve any pressure on the heart when hypotension occurs.

Intraoperative Concerns for Robotic Thymectomy

The initial decision during robotic mediastinal resection is whether to approach the dissection from the left chest, right chest, or bilaterally. Often this decision is dictated by the anatomy of the lesion. The right-sided approach offers superior visualization and operative space, owing to the predominance of the heart in the left chest. Further, it offers direct visualization of the superior vena cava, innominate vein, and the origin of the right internal mammary vessels. These structures serve as important landmarks for superior mediastinal dissection during thymectomy.

We have observed, however, that resection of the thymic horns is often easier from the left chest (**Fig. 6**). Additionally, rests of thymic tissue are more commonly found under the left aspect of the innominate vein in the superior mediastinum and in the aortopulmonary window, both of which are often difficult to access from the right chest. From a surgical standpoint, we prefer the left-sided approach to thymectomy in patients with myasthenia gravis or thymoma, given that completeness of resection is the only factor predictive of long-term survival for thymoma and for durable decrease of symptoms in patients with myasthenia gravis.

Preservation of the bilateral phrenic nerves during mediastinal robotic surgery is critical to prevent diaphragmatic dysfunction or paralysis. Observation of the contralateral nerve is facilitated with the use of a 30° camera and decreasing the insufflation of carbon dioxide, which brings the pericardium into the anterior mediastinum. In cases where the phrenic nerves cannot be easily located,

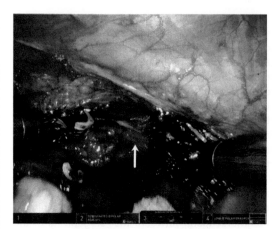

Fig. 6. Dissection of the right superior thymic horn (*arrow*) during left-sided robotic thymectomy.

ICG can be administered intravenously to illuminate the phrenic veins which flank the nerves. Last, an additional trocar can be placed in the contralateral chest to view the nerve via thoracoscopy.

In patients without myasthenia gravis, if the mediastinal lesion involves the phrenic nerve, one of the nerves can be sacrificed to achieve a complete resection, but not both. If a complete resection cannot be achieved, or if both nerves are involved, a reductive surgery is performed. If a phrenic nerve is inadvertently transected, primary suture repair of the nerve can be attempted. In cases of phrenic nerve transection, we do not recommend immediate diaphragmatic plication, because postoperative function remains unknown and the diaphragm lacks redundancy, making plication difficult.

Injury to the innominate vein, which is often obscured by mediastinal fat and the thymus, may occur during dissection into the superior mediastinum. Smaller injuries may be controlled with pressure from a rolled up sponge. Topical hemostatic agents can be used for continued oozing or limited bleeding. More significant injuries may require packing to obtain hemostatic control, allowing time for conversion to an open sternotomy to repair the injury directly.

ROBOTIC ESOPHAGECTOMY

Minimally invasive esophagectomy has demonstrated superior short-term postoperative outcomes versus open esophagectomy. In a prospective randomized comparison of open versus robotic esophagectomy, a robotic approach was associated with lower immediate posterior pain and decreased incidence of pulmonary complications.[16] Long-term oncologic

outcomes specific to robotic esophagectomy are not well described and remain a focus on ongoing investigation. Interestingly, lymph node resection has been shown to be greater with a robotic approach, potentially leading to more accurate staging and/or extended survival.

Anesthetic Considerations

For robotic esophagectomy, an arterial line and urinary catheter are placed given the anticipated length of the procedure and possibility of hemodynamic change. A single lumen endotracheal tube is placed initially for the abdominal portion of the procedure and then exchanged for a double lumen tube for the thoracic phase of the operation. Initially using a single-lumen tube decreases the amount of time that the patient has a larger diameter double lumen tube in place.

Management of the Pylorus

During esophagectomy with gastric pull-up, the bilateral vagus nerves are transected, leaving patients susceptible to gastric emptying complications. The addition of a pyloric emptying procedure during esophagectomy aims to limit the sequelae of vagotomy. The optimal management of the pylorus—no intervention, endoscopic dilation, botulinum toxin injection, pyloromotomy, or pyloroplasty—remains controversial. In a retrospective review comparing pyloric interventions during esophagectomy, the omission of an emptying procedure resulted in a greater incidence of aspiration.[17] Further, the functional outcomes and complication profile of botulinum toxin injection were similar to more invasive interventions. Our procedure of choice is injection of botulinum toxin at the pylorus. If postoperative emptying is abnormal, we perform endoscopy with balloon dilation of the pylorus.

Gastroesophageal Anastomosis

The gastroesophageal anastomosis can be completely hand sewn, completely stapled (linear or circular stapler), or a combination of the 2 methods (a linear stapler for the posterior wall and a hand sewn anterior wall). The optimal approach to performing the anastomosis is a matter of debate. We have observed that a completely stapled anastomoses results in a higher rate of stricture. We prefer a linear stapled posterior anastomosis with a hand sewn anterior portion.

The gastric conduit must be aligned appropriately, without twisting or tension. A gastrotomy is made in the posterior wall of the conduit at least 2 cm proximal to the tip of the conduit and distant from the staple line. The remaining anterior wall of the anastomosis is closed using a running barbed locking suture. The anastomosis should be inspected, and any questionable areas should have repair sutures placed. Endoscopy can be performed, and the integrity of the anastomosis checked via air insufflation while submerged in saline. Preserving an omental flap during the abdominal phase allows for wrapping of the anastomosis, which protects the adjacent airway and decreases the risk of anastomotic leak.

Assessment of tissue perfusion can help determine the viability of the gastroesophageal anastomosis. Intravenous injection of ICG contrast illuminates perfused tissue, revealing the optimal area of transection of the conduit for anastomosis (**Fig. 7**). Investigators have described a 0% leak rate in 39 cases after instituting routine perfusion assessment using ICG to guide creation of the esophagotomy and performance of the gastroesophageal anastomosis.[18] The use of ICG and near-infrared fluorescence imaging can also help with assessment of the vascular arcade during mobilization of the gastric conduit during the abdominal phase of the operation.

CONVERSION TO OPEN THORACOTOMY

A significant intraoperative decision in robotic surgery is deciding when to abandon a minimally invasive approach and convert to an open thoracotomy. Conversion to thoracotomy sacrifices the advantages of minimally invasive surgery and contributes to increased postoperative pain, length of stay, and pulmonary complications. Conversion, however, may become the safest way to proceed after particular intraoperative challenges and complications. The conversion rate for robotic surgery and VATS are similar, ranging from 2% to 10% in institutional series.[19] The decision for

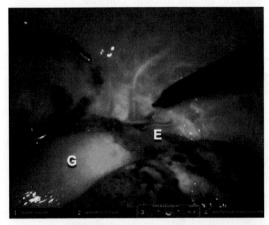

Fig. 7. Visualization of tissue perfusion of the neoesophageal anastomosis using ICG contrast. E, esophagus; G, gastric conduit.

conversion to thoracotomy is either the result of an intraoperative complication and/or failure of the minimally invasive approach. The timing of the decision largely depends on a surgeon's experience and the patient's clinical status.

One of the primary reasons for conversion to thoracotomy is when exposure cannot be established safely, most commonly owing to severe pleural adhesions preventing the placement of the robotic ports. Moderate adhesions, such as those encountered in early pleural empyema, can typically be taken down with sweeping of the robotic camera or drainage of pleural fluid with sequential placement of the ports as pleural space is created.

Surgeons may also elect to convert to open thoracotomy to ameliorate frustration during difficult or unusually lengthy cases. Intraoperative challenges such as dissection of dense hilar lymph nodes adherent to pulmonary vessels or a hostile fissure can lead surgeons to convert to an open approach. In a retrospective review of patients undergoing pulmonary resection after neoadjuvant nivolumab, 13 patients underwent minimally invasive resection, of which 7 (54%) required thoracotomy.[20] The authors reported that operative notes in these patients noted dense, vascularized chest all adhesions, and/or dense adhesions in the fissure.

Intraoperative complications, such as hemorrhage, injury to the diaphragm, airway injury, or injury to abdominal organs such as the spleen or liver, may also prompt surgeons to open thoracotomy. Although complications may occur, surgeons must be aware of the potential for problems, anticipate them, and be prepared to address them expeditiously.

Pulmonary Vascular Injury

Given the intimate relationship of the hilar structures in the chest and potential for anatomic variation, thoracic surgeons must be prepared for injury to vascular structures. The pulmonary arteries and pulmonary veins may be injured from a number of mechanisms, including excessive retraction or tearing of a vessel, direct injury during dissection, stapler malfunction, or injury during dissection of an adherent adjacent structure (such as a lymph node or a bronchus). Dark pulsatile bleeding is suggestive of an injury to the pulmonary artery, which occurs in 0.5% to 3.0% of minimally invasive pulmonary lobectomies.[18]

In a multi-institutional series assessing for intraoperative catastrophes during robotic pulmonary resection, 35 events were found among 1810 cases, with conversion to thoracotomy in 31 (89%).[21] An intraoperative catastrophe was defined as any circumstance leading to an emergency thoracotomy after robotic docking and/or requiring an additional major surgical procedure. As expected, risk factors for catastrophic events included higher tumor stage and higher patient comorbidity status. Equally, catastrophic events were associated with increased length of stay, postoperative complications, and mortality. The most common catastrophic event was intraoperative hemorrhage owing to injury of the pulmonary artery or pulmonary vein, with such injuries most commonly occurring in the context of adherent hilar lymphadenopathy. Vascular injury was most common during left upper lobectomy, representing 35% of cases. Importantly, bleeding from the pulmonary artery led to intraoperative death in 2 patients.

Given the gravity of an intraoperative vascular injury during robotic pulmonary resection, it is critical for operating teams to be prepared for major hemorrhage. Our strategy for managing bleeding from a major vessel injury can be summarized as the 4 Ps: poise, pressure, preparedness, and proximal control. Pressure is applied to the site of vessel injury with a rolled-up sponge (**Fig. 8**). Meanwhile, the anesthesia team and nurses prepare for a possible thoracotomy, and other experienced surgeons are called for assistance as necessary. If possible, proximal control of the bleeding vessel is obtained. The vessel can then be divided with a stapler or the distal injury repaired directly with suture.

Although rare in overall incidence, intraoperative catastrophic events represent critical instances that particularly highlight the value of thorough preparation and robust communication among members of the robotic surgical team.

Airway Injury

Injury to a noninvolved (not divided during the operation) airway, either the proximal trachea, or a distal segmental bronchus, is rare. The most common mechanism of airway injury, however, is a posterior membranous tear from a forceful or oversized double-lumen endotracheal tube. During pulmonary lobectomy, injury to the left or right mainstem airways may occur during dissection of the station 7 lymph nodes or the distal trachea during resection of the station 4 lymph nodes (**Fig. 9**). The use of bipolar cautery decreases the likelihood of thermal injury during dissection of lymph nodes. Airway injury often requires a reconfiguration of airway control, with advancement beyond the defect if possible. Buttressed repair or segmental resection with reconstruction is often required. Mobilization of mediastinal fat, pleural patch, or intercostal muscle are optional adjuncts to place over the site of airway repair.

OPERATIVE EFFICIENCY AND TEACHING

As hospitals and care systems continue to promote value-based care and bundled payments, physicians and surgeons are tasked to optimize value at every stage of patient care. From an operative perspective, we have found that, regardless of the approach (open vs minimally invasive), total operative time is a surrogate for outcomes. We retrospectively reviewed the Premier Healthcare Database for patients undergoing elective pulmonary lobectomy and found that 15-minute incremental increases beyond an operative time of 3 hours were associated with longer lengths of stay (0.12 days) higher costs (total cost $893, operative costs $376, and nonoperative costs $516), more in-hospital complications (odds ratio, 1.05), and increased 30-day readmission rates (odds ratio, 1.02).[22] We believe that the correlation between total operative time and value may be a surrogate marker of surgical competence, teamwork, and efficiency.

Teaching on the Robotic Console

Despite an exacting health care environment focused on perioperative metrics such as patient

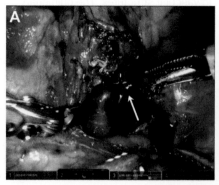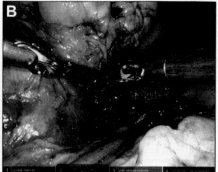

Fig. 8. Intraoperative injury to a pulmonary artery. (*A*) Bleeding from a pulmonary artery branch in the left upper lobe (*arrow*). (*B*) Robotic hemostatic control with application of pressure with a sponge.

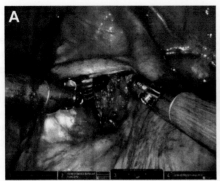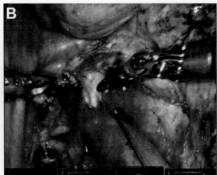

Fig. 9. Robotic lymph node resection. (*A*) Station 4 lymph node resection, with dissection underneath the azygos vein, adjacent the trachea. (*B*) Station 7 lymph node resection with visualization of the left mainstem bronchus.

satisfaction and outcomes, it is incumbent on thoracic surgeons to teach residents how to safely and efficiently perform minimally invasive thoracic surgery. On the robotic system, a second optional console allows for tandem surgery, permitting a clear field of view and fluid instrument exchange for a second surgeon or trainee. Unique to the robotic system, the trainee's operative field and instruments are in the exact orientation and perspective as the primary surgeon. Owing in part to this technology, the operative conduct of robotic surgery can be taught without compromising patient outcomes.[23] For pulmonary lobectomy, we break down the operation into a series of defined steps. Typically, trainees start by mastering dissection of the lymph node stations, then progress to higher risk maneuvers such as robotic stapling and pulmonary artery dissection. Further, video recording of the operation can be easily saved on the robotic system, for later review and analysis of technique.

REFERENCES

1. Hemmerling TM, Schmidt J, Bosert C, et al. Systemic air embolism during wedge resection of the lung. Anesth Analg 2001;93(5):1135.
2. Baldini G, Bagry H, Aprikian A, et al. Postoperative urinary retention: anesthetic and perioperative considerations. Anesthesiology 2009;110(5):1139–57.
3. Kehlet H, Wilmore DW. Multimodal strategies to improve surgical outcome. Am J Surg 2002;183(6):630–41.
4. King NM, Quiko AS, Slotto JG, et al. Retrospective analysis of quality improvement when using liposomal bupivacaine for postoperative pain control. J Pain Res 2016;9:233–40.
5. Khalil KG, Boutrous ML, Irani AD, et al. Operative intercostal nerve blocks with long-acting bupivacaine liposome for pain control after thoracotomy. Ann Thorac Surg 2015;100:2013–8.
6. Lee CY, Robinson DA, Johnson CA, et al. A randomized controlled trial of liposomal bupivacaine parasternal intercostal block for sternotomy. Ann Thorac Surg 2019;107:128–34.
7. Grichnik K, Clark J. Pathophysiology and management of one-lung ventilation. Thorac Surg Clin 2005;15(1):84–103.
8. Kent M, Wang T, Whyte R, et al. Open, video-assisted thoracic surgery, and robotic lobectomy: review of a national database. Ann Thorac Surg 2014;97:236–42.
9. Cerfolio RJ, Ghanim AF, Dylewski M, et al. The long-term survival of robotic lobectomy for non-small cell lung cancer: a multi-institutional study. J Thorac Cardiovasc Surg 2018;155:778–86.
10. Geraci TC, Ferrari-Light D, Kent A, et al. Technique, outcomes with navigational bronchoscopy using indocyanine green for robotic segmentectomy. Ann Thorac Surg 2019;108(2):363–9.
11. Kodama K, Higashiyama M, Okami J, et al. Oncologic outcomes of segmentectomy versus lobectomy for clinical T1aN0M0 non-small cell lung cancer. Ann Thorac Surg 2016;101(2):504–11.
12. Asamura H. Role of limited sublobar resection for early-stage lung cancer: steady progress. J Clin Oncol 2014;32:2403–4.
13. Clark F. Reduction of intraoperative air leaks with Progel in pulmonary resection: a comprehensive review. J Cardiothorac Surg 2013;8:90.
14. Brunelli A, Sabbatini A, Xiume' F, et al. Alternate suction reduces prolonged air leak after pulmonary lobectomy: a randomized comparison versus water seal. Ann Thorac Surg 2005;80(3):1052–5.
15. Cerfolio RJ, Minnich DJ, Bryant AS. The removal of chest tubes despite an air leak or a pneumothorax. Ann Thorac Surg 2009;87(6):1690–6.
16. Sarkaria IS, Rizk NP, Goldman DA, et al. Early quality of life outcomes after robotic-assisted minimally invasive and open esophagectomy. Ann Thorac Surg 2019;108:920–8.

17. Antonoff MB, Puri V, Meyers BF, et al. Comparison of pyloric intervention strategies at the time of esophagectomy: is more better? Ann Thorac Surg 2014; 97(6):1950–8.

18. Hodari A, Park KU, Lace B, et al. Robot-assisted minimally invasive Ivor Lewis esophagectomy with real-time perfusion assessment. Ann Thorac Surg 2015;100:947–52.

19. Brian L. Catastrophes and complicated intraoperative events during robotic lung resection. J Vis Surg 2017;3:52.

20. Bott MJ, Yang SC, Park BJ, et al. Initial results of pulmonary resection after neoadjuvant nivolumab in patients with resectable non-small cell lung cancer. J Thorac Cardiovasc Surg 2019;158(1): 269–76.

21. Cao C, Cerfolio RJ, Louie BE, et al. Incidence, management and outcomes of intraoperative catastrophes during robotic pulmonary resection. Ann Thorac Surg 2019;108(5):1498–504.

22. Ferrari-Light D, Geraci TC, Cerfolio RJ. Prolonged operative time for pulmonary lobectomy predicts worse outcomes and lower value. Abstract presentation #50 at the Southern Thoracic Surgical Association 66th Annual Meeting on November 8, 2019 in Marco Island, FL.

23. Cerfolio RJ, Cichos KH, Wei B, et al. Robotic lobectomy can be taught while maintaining quality patient outcomes. J Thorac Cardiovasc Surg 2016;152(4):991–7.

Prevention of Postoperative Prolonged Air Leak After Pulmonary Resection

Praveen Sridhar, MD[a], Virginia R. Litle, MD[b], Morihito Okada, MD PhD[c], Kei Suzuki, MD[b],*

KEYWORDS

- Postoperative air leak • Pulmonary resection • Pleural patch • Pleural tent • Pleural sealant
- Prophylactic pneumoperitoneum

KEY POINTS

- There is no gold standard for the prevention of postoperative air leaks after thoracic surgery.
- In patients with intraoperative air leaks, use of polyglycolic acid mesh and sealants is safe and may decrease the duration of air leak, chest drainage, and hospital stay.
- Pleural tenting is a useful tool for the prevention of air leak in upper lobectomies.
- There is no standard management for postoperative tube thoracostomy, although, conditionally, the use of continued suction is not superior to water seal in reducing the duration of air leak.

INTRODUCTION

Postoperative prolonged air leaks (PALs) occur after thoracic surgery, most often in patients undergoing either oncologic lung resection or lung volume reduction surgery (LVRS).[1–4] Air leaks occur via parenchymal defects, preventing sealing of the pleural space after resection.[3] Between 8% and 26% of patients who undergo lobectomies and up to 46% of patients undergoing LVRS have PALs.[3]

Although PALs can be managed in multiple ways, the sequelae of these leaks are increased intensive care unit readmissions, longer hospital stays, a higher incidence of pneumonia, and pleural space infections.[3] Historically, the management of PALs following thoracic surgery has been limited to watchful waiting with continued tube thoracostomy for drainage.[3] PALs secondary to alveolar-pleural fistulas rather than bronchopleural fistulas are likely to resolve over time with expectant management, although some controversy exists with regard to chest tube management.[5–8] In addition, the use of 1-way valves averts the need for prolonged hospital stays for patients who can tolerate water sealing of their chest tubes.[2]

Although there are several methods that have been used to treat PALs after they are diagnosed, populations at risk for developing an air leak have been identified and prophylactic measures can be

a Division of Thoracic Surgery, Department of Surgery, Boston Medical Center, Boston University School of Medicine, Surgical Education Office, 88 East Newton Street, Collamore Building, Suite C-515, Boston, MA 02118, USA; b Division of Thoracic Surgery, Department of Surgery, Boston Medical Center, Boston University School of Medicine, Boston University, 88 East Newton Street, Collamore Building, Suite 7380, Boston, MA 02118, USA; c Department of Surgical Oncology, Hiroshima University, 1-2-3 Kasumi, Minami-ku, Hiroshima City, Hiroshima 734-8551, Japan
* Corresponding author.
E-mail address: Kei.Suzuki@bmc.org
Twitter: @Psridhar127 (P.S.); @vlitlemd (V.R.L.)

Thorac Surg Clin 30 (2020) 305–314
https://doi.org/10.1016/j.thorsurg.2020.04.007
1547-4127/20/© 2020 Elsevier Inc. All rights reserved.

taken at the index operation to prevent the onset of PALs. Female patients or those with chronic obstructive pulmonary disease, low forced expiratory volume in 1 second (FEV_1), a smoking history, diabetes, or chronic steroid use have been identified as high risk for developing PAL following lobectomy. Patients undergoing LVRS who have low diffusing capacity of the lungs for carbon monoxide and FEV_1, pleural adhesions, or diffuse emphysema are also more prone to develop PALs.[3] This article discusses the several prophylactic measures that have been studied for the prevention of PALs following lung resection, including the use of absorbable mesh, parenchymal sealants, pleural tenting, staple line buttresses, and prophylactic pneumoperitoneum.

PLEURAL MESH PATCH

The use of polyglycolic acid (PGA) mesh sheets for the coverage of pulmonary parenchyma has been studied in various contexts[9–23] (**Table 1**). Nakamura and colleagues[19] evaluated the safety of PGA staple line buttress as well as PGA mesh coverage for stapled, sutured, and unsutured parenchyma following sublobar and lobar resections in a cohort of 344 of 1026 patients. No additional sealant was added, and there were no differences in surgical site infectious complications between patients with and without mesh use. Yoshimoto and colleagues[22] examined mesh coverage of the parenchyma compared with suture closure of the visceral pleura in the setting of segmental resection. The purpose of mesh coverage of the parenchyma was to augment the benefit of lung

preservation provided by performing sublobar resection; however, transection of the parenchyma resulted in exposed raw lung surface that predisposed patients to PAL. Although suture closure of the pleura had conventionally been used, this theoretically reduced lung expansion. Therefore, the utility of the PGA sheet was to cover the intersegmental plane, minimize PAL, and maximize lung function relative to suture closure. Although this study did not reveal a difference in postoperative lung function, it was not designed to compare PAL in mesh versus nonmesh coverage.

Since these initial studies, the utility of PGA mesh coverage for the prevention of PAL has been studied alone and in combination with other closure techniques for coverage of raw parenchymal surfaces following oncologic resection as well as lung resection for benign disease (**Fig. 1**). Saito and colleagues[13] reexamined the use of PGA mesh in addition to fibrin glue to prevent pulmonary complications after segmental resection for stage IA non–small cell lung cancer in a case-control study. Although the investigators confirmed no differences in pulmonary function for up to 6 months postoperatively, they noted an increased incidence of PAL associated with mesh use compared with suture closure of the pleura on univariate (8.7% vs 0%; $P = .042$) and regression analysis (odds ratio, 5.26; $P = .047$).[13]

Okada and colleagues[18] routinely used a PGA patch in combination with a fibrin sealant to cover the intersegmental plane following thermal dissection during segmentectomy, as described in a series of 52 patients who underwent segmentectomy

Table 1
Polyglycolic acid mesh pneumostasis for patients undergoing lung resection

Author, Year	Study Design (n)	Dissection and Closure	Duration Chest Tube Drainage			Mean Length of Stay (d)		
			Mesh	No Mesh	P Value	Mesh	No Mesh	P Value
Ueda et al,[14] 2007	Prospective (45)	Stapler PGA mesh Fibrin	1[d]	1.2	.205	6.8	7.1	.694
Ueda et al,[23] 2010	Retrospective (122)	Stapler PGA mesh[a] Fibrin	1[c]	2	<.001	8.7	11	.007
Saito et al,[13] 2017	Retrospective (133)	Cautery[b] PGA mesh Fibrin	7.5[d]	4.1	<.001	15.7	10.2	<.001

[a] Control group treated with fibrin glue alone compared with mesh plus fibrin glue.
[b] Control group with pleural suture closure alone.
[c] Median number of days.
[d] Mean number of days.

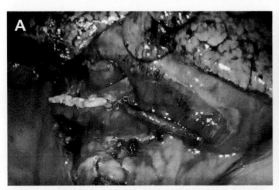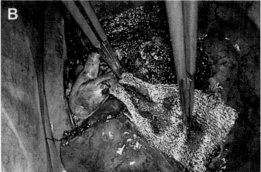

Fig. 1. Application of PGA mesh sheet to staple line after fibrin application. (*A*) Fibrin applied endoscopically to staple line via spray. (*B*) Mesh situated over staple line or over divided parenchyma.

for stage I cancers. There were 4 PALs (7.7%), with a 1-day median duration for all air leaks and thoracostomy drainage for a median 3 days for all patients. Kawai and colleagues[9] applied low-voltage energy as well as PGA mesh and fibrin sealant to pleural defects in 40 patients with an intraoperative air leak out of a total cohort of 176 who had undergone thoracoscopic lobectomy for neoplasm. They compared patients with energy, mesh, and fibrin with those without intraoperative leaks for whom only mesh and fibrin were used. Intraoperative air leaks were defined as air leakage with a −20 cm H_2O pressure load. Air leaks resolved in nearly 80% of patients and, for those with postoperative air leaks, no patients had leaks >7 days (median 3.5 days). Note that patients with intraoperative air leaks required 3 more days of chest drainage compared with those without intraoperative air leaks (5.3 days vs 2.2 days). These data suggested a possible utility for mesh pneumostasis in patients with an intraoperative air leak; however, this method of pneumostasis did not entirely avert the need for prolonged chest drainage.

Ueda and colleagues[14,16,23] addressed this in a series of studies on patients with intraoperative air leaks discovered on intraoperative water-seal tests following resection for neoplastic disease. Ueda and colleagues[14] attempted to prevent postoperative air leaks by identifying leaks intraoperatively and applying a fibrin sealant–soaked PGA mesh in 28 patients compared with 17 patients who had no intraoperative leak and were consequently not treated with mesh or sealant. There was no significant difference in the duration of chest drainage in patients who underwent mesh and fibrin closure relative to those who did not, and all intraoperative air leaks resolved immediately. Two patients developed delayed air leaks requiring redrainage. A follow-up study by Ueda and colleagues[16] described results for 133

patients with intraoperative air leaks who underwent mesh and fibrin pneumostasis compared with 73 with no intraoperative air leak and no mesh pneumostasis. Similar to the initial study, delayed pneumothorax occurred in treated patients (3%) requiring redrainage, but there was no difference in median chest tube duration between those with and without an intraoperative air leak. Importantly, Ueda and colleagues[23] described a safe and effective method of prophylactic mesh and fibrin application; however, these studies did not offer a direct comparison of mesh versus no mesh pneumostasis, because intraoperative air leaks may not have been clinically significant if left untreated. A separate study of 145 patients with intraoperative air leaks who underwent fibrin alone compared with mesh plus fibrin closure did reveal that patients with mesh and fibrin pneumostasis had 1 fewer day of chest tube drainage as well as a shorter hospital stay.

Lee and colleagues[12] applied the use of PGA mesh pneumostasis for patients undergoing bullectomy and mechanical pleurodesis for spontaneous pneumothoraces. Notably in patients who underwent bullectomy, pleurodesis, and PGA mesh pneumostasis, there was a higher recurrence-free rate over a 24-month follow-up period (94.9% PGA mesh vs 89% no mesh; log-rank $P = .047$). Although 4 patients treated without PGA mesh pneumostasis required reoperation for recurrent pneumothoraces, all patients with recurrences following mesh pneumostasis were successfully treated nonoperatively. Saito and colleagues[17] followed 11 patients after bullectomy with PGA mesh staple line reinforcement for a median of 11 months with no air leaks postoperatively and no recurrent pneumothoraces. Hirai and colleagues[21] retrospectively reviewed 173 patients treated with bullectomy and PGA mesh and fibrin coverage to reinforce staple line pneumostasis and found that only 3% of patients had recurrent pneumothorax compared with almost a 20% recurrence rate in patients treated during the same period with only stapling.

Although these data for pleural patch pneumostasis in combination with several other techniques for closure are compelling, there have been no trials in the United States prospectively examining the role for prophylactic mesh pneumostasis in any patients undergoing open or thoracoscopic lung resection.

SEALANTS
Polyethylene Glycol Hydrogel

Several sealants have been studied, including homologous and autologous fibrin-based sealants, and polyethylene glycol (PEG)–based absorbable sealants. This article reviews both fibrin-based and PEG-based sealants, because these have been studied extensively for the treatment of intraoperative air leak and the prevention of PALs (**Table 2**).[24–36] Although there are multiple formulations of homologous fibrin-based sealants, these are generally composed of human fibrinogen and thrombin.[33–36] Autologous fibrin-based sealants are generated from patient blood samples taken intraoperatively.[32]

The efficacy of a biodegradable polymer was established by Allen and colleagues[25] in a multicenter prospective randomized controlled trial in which patients undergoing open resection for both benign and malignant disease underwent randomization following the identification of intraoperative air leaks to PEG-based pneumostasis or

Table 2
Sealants for pneumostasis for patients undergoing lung resection

Author, Year	Study Design (n)	Experimental Technique	Duration Chest Tube Drainage			Mean Length of Stay (d)		
			Sealant	No Sealant	P Value	Sealant	No Sealant	P Value
Allen et al,[24] 2004	Prospective (148)	PEG	6.8[b]	6.2	.679	6[a]	7	.028
Anegg et al,[33] 2007	Prospective (152)	Homologous fibrin	5.1[b]	6.3	.022	6.2	7.7	.01
Rena et al,[36] 2009	Prospective (50)	Homologous fibrin	3.5[b]	5.9	.002	5.9	7.5	.01
Dango et al,[30] 2010	Retrospective (40)	PEG	2.1[a]	3.9	.030	9.9	11.7	.178
Gonfiotti et al,[35] 2011	Prospective (185)	Homologous fibrin	5.96[b]	6.54	.992	7.64	7.58	.712
Tan et al,[28] 2011	Prospective (119)	PEG	4[a]	3	NR	7[a]	6	NR
Lequaglie et al,[27] 2012	Prospective (222)	PEG	—	—	—	4.3	8.4	.0001
Filosso et al,[34] 2013	Prospective (24)	Homologous fibrin	6.1[b]	10.8	<.001	6.9	9.5	<.001
Gologorsky et al,[29] 2019	Retrospective (176)	PEG	1[a]	1	.721	—	—	—

Abbreviation: NR, not reported.
[a] Median number of days.
[b] Mean number of days.

no further pneumostasis. Intraoperative air leak was defined by the presence of air bubbles greater than or equal to 2 mm with lung inflation to 20 to 25 cm H_2O after pulmonary resection. Following assessment for intraoperative air leaks, randomized patients underwent conventional methods of air leak control (suture or staple) compared with these methods plus application of reconstituted sealant. The incidence of PALs and duration of chest tube drainage were not different between the 2 groups despite the decrease in perioperative air leaks in patients following sealant application. Park and colleagues[26] established that PEG hydrogel was safe with similar outcomes for air leakage and chest tube drainage primarily in robotic and video-assisted thoracoscopy.

A smaller case-matched retrospective cohort study by Dango and colleagues[30] of 40 patients revealed a shorter time to chest tube removal for patients with sealant application relative to those without sealant. Although the investigators report that the limiting factor accounting for this difference was the presence of an air leak, all patients had 2 surgical chest tubes placed for drainage, and the time to discontinuation of the second chest tube did not significantly differ. Tan and colleagues[28] conducted a similarly sized study that failed to show any significant differences in patients with intraoperative air leaks randomized to no therapy versus PEG-based hydrogel application. Intraoperative air leaks were assessed after inflation of the lung to 25 cm H_2O.

Although these studies did not show compelling evidence for or against the use of hydrogel sealants, multiple prospective studies have shown some benefit. Data from a single-center, prospective trial of 222 randomized patients undergoing open or minimally invasive resection for benign and malignant tumors by Lequaglie and colleagues[27] suggested that sealants reduced the percentage of patients with air leaks more than 5 days (2.7% vs 11.4%; $P = .0013$) as well as the mean length of hospital stay (4.3 days vs 8.4 days; $P = .0001$). D'Andrilli and colleagues[31] used a different PEG-based Biogel sealant in a prospective randomized trial for open anatomic and nonanatomic resections. Similar to previous studies, patients were randomized intraoperatively after air leak was identified. An important difference in this study was the use of buttressed staple lines with bovine pericardium in all patients. D'Andrilli and colleagues[31] found not only that perioperative air leaks were more likely to resolve in the sealant group but that the total duration of air leak was shorter in the sealant group relative to standard closure (3.5 days vs 4.2 days; $P = .01$).

Homologous and Autologous Fibrin Sealants

Homologous human fibrinogen and thrombin has been approved for the closure of alveolar air leaks following lung resection and subsequently has been evaluated for its efficacy in several studies.[33–36] Anegg and colleagues[33] initially published a single-center, prospective, randomized trial in which patients underwent anatomic resection for cancer. The investigators included patients with mild to moderate intraoperative air leak measured via spirometry by the anesthesiologist as lungs were inflated to 25 cm H_2O. These patients were then randomized to the use of a fibrin sealant patch or to no additional pneumostasis. Severe air leaks were treated with pledget-reinforced parenchymal suturing and were randomized on leak retesting. Although the rate of prolonged air leak greater than 7 days was not significantly different, patients with fibrin closure had a mean time to chest tube removal that was approximately 1 day shorter than nonreinforced closure and were consequently discharged 1 day earlier.

Rena and colleagues[36] importantly assessed the efficacy of fibrin patch and cautery-assisted pneumostasis in patients with incomplete or absent fissures undergoing lobectomy compared with stapled fissural development alone. Prolonged air leak greater than 7 days was associated with standard stapled development of the fissure compared with fibrin-assisted closure (26.7% vs 3.3%; $P = .029$). The durations of chest tube drainage (3.5 days vs 5.9 days; $P = .002$) and hospital stay (5.9 days vs 7.5 days; $P = .01$) were also reduced in patients who had fibrin patch–assisted closure.[36]

Gonfiotti and colleagues[35] conducted a well-designed prospective trial that was adequately powered to show a reduction in duration of air leak in patients undergoing lung resection. Study surgeons across multiple institutions used uniform resection techniques with stapled development of fissural planes. Patients were randomized after diagnosis and grading of intraoperative air leaks to either fibrin sealant pneumostasis or no further therapy. The duration of postoperative air leak in patients with fibrin sealant pneumostasis was significantly lower (43 hours vs 67 hours; $P<.005$), although the duration of chest tube drainage and the length of hospital stay was not.[35]

In addition, a study by Moser and colleagues[32] is worth mention. Although limited by small sample size (25 patients), the investigators performed bilateral thoracoscopic LVRS for emphysema and were consequently uniquely positioned to perform a case-control study in which 1 lung was treated with autologous fibrin sealant pneumostasis, but the contralateral lung was not. Prolonged air leak greater than 7 days was noted in only 1 (4.5% PAL) lung treated with fibrin sealant, whereas 7 lungs (31.8%) without fibrin pneumostasis experienced PAL (P = .031). In addition, 2 of the nontreated lungs required reoperation.[32]

PLEURAL TENTING

Unlike patching or applying fibrin sealants, pleural tenting does not entail the use of a foreign body to achieve pneumostasis. The technique of pleural tenting involves dissection of the parietal pleura at the superior and lateral thoracic cavity and separating this layer from the endothoracic fascia apically and medially to the mediastinal pleura, followed by suturing the free edge of the dissected pleura to an intercostal space adjacent to the remaining lung parenchyma.[37] This technique allows prevention of air leaks by pleural apposition without full lung expansion into the residual resection cavity. Although there are fewer studies examining the role of pleural tenting as opposed to sealant or mesh use, data regarding the use of pleural tenting following upper lobectomies have been encouraging.[37–42]

Allama and colleagues,[37] Brunelli and colleagues,[42] Okur and colleagues,[40] and Robinson and colleagues[39] conducted studies on patients undergoing upper lobectomy or bilobectomy with pleural tenting, showing an association between this technique and decreased duration of postoperative air leak (**Table 3**). The earliest studies conducted by Robinson and colleagues[39] and Okur and colleagues[40] completed in the late 1990s on small cohorts of fewer than 50 patients undergoing upper lobectomies or bilobectomies revealed shorter durations of air leaks and chest tube drainage in the tented groups. Brunelli and colleagues[42] prospectively performed the largest study on a cohort of 200 patients undergoing upper lobectomies or bilobectomies, of whom 100

were randomized to additional pleural tenting. All patients underwent thoracotomy and staplers were used for parenchymal division. Patients who underwent pleural tenting had an air leak for a mean of 2.5 days compared with 7.2 days without tenting (P<.0001) and had chest tube drainage for 7 days compared with 11.2 days (P<.0001). Although these differences are remarkable, the rate of prolonged air leak greater than 7 days was noted in almost half of patents without pleural tenting compared with about 16% in patients undergoing pleural tenting. Although the rate of prolonged air leak in patients who received tenting was similar to other published data of patients undergoing lung resection, the rate in those without tenting was drastically higher than in contemporary reports.[3,42]

Allama and colleagues[37] then prospectively studied 48 patients in a randomized trial, of whom 23 received pleural tenting for upper or right bilobectomies, with the duration of air leak and the presence of a prolonged air leak greater than 5 days being significantly lower in the tent group relative to the nontent group. Despite this, the duration of chest tube drainage was not significantly different.

PROPHYLACTIC PNEUMOPERITONEUM

Just as pleural tenting can be an effective strategy to avoid PALs in upper and right bilobectomies, prophylactic pneumoperitoneum has been studied as a method to avoid this complication in right lower and lower bilobectomies.[43–45] There are few studies that have evaluated therapeutic pneumoperitoneum at the time of the index operation with fewer than 100 patients described in the literature.[43–45] Despite this small sample size, the 2 prospective, double-armed trials did show that patients with prophylactic pneumoperitoneum had significantly fewer incidences of PALs greater than 5 days, a shorter duration of chest tube drainage, and shorter hospital stays.[43,44]

Table 3
Pleural tent for pneumostasis for patients undergoing lung resection

Author, Year	Study Design (n)	Mean Duration Chest Tube Drainage (d)			Mean Length of Stay (d)		
		Tent	No Tent	P Value	Tent	No Tent	P Value
Robinson & Preksto,[39] 1997	Retrospective (48)	4	6.6	.004	6.4	8.6	.02
Okur et al,[40] 2001	Prospective (40)	4.3	7.4	<.0001	7.6	9.3	.024
Brunelli et al,[42] 2002	Prospective (200)	7	11.2	<.0001	8.2	11.6	<.0001
Allama et al,[37] 2010	Prospective (48)	4.6	5.6	.11	4.96	5.70	.05

Okur and colleagues[44] prospectively studied 60 patients, 30 of whom were randomized to receive intraoperative prophylactic pneumoperitoneum with 1 to 1.5 L of room air via a right-sided trans-diaphragmatic catheter. All patients in both arms underwent intraoperative leak testing and suture repair of parenchymal leaks before additional intervention. Patients with pneumoperitoneum had a mean chest tube duration of 3.47 days compared with 4.87 days ($P<.001$) for those without pneumoperitoneum, and only 1 patient had a prolonged air leak greater than 5 days in the pneumoperitoneum group compared with the control group ($P = .026$).

STAPLE LINE BUTTRESS

Staple line buttressing has commonly been used for prophylaxis against parenchymal staple line air leaks in lung resection.[46–48] A variety of buttresses have been tested in this setting, including bovine pericardium, expanded polytetrafluoro-ethylene, and PGA.[48] Takamochi and colleagues[48] performed a recent prospective study of 41 patients undergoing a lobectomy for benign and neoplastic disease using PGA sheets to staple lines compared with 35 patients without a buttress. The data gathered from this study are difficult to interpret because more than half of the patients in both groups had additional sealant or suturing for intraoperative air leaks. Regardless, there was no significant difference in the duration of air leak or the duration of chest drain placement.

One aspect of postoperative air leak management that is variable across nearly every study and study method is postoperative chest tube management. Drahush and colleagues[46] not only performed a buttressed closure with extracellular mesh strips but used protocolized postoperative chest tube management and a fissureless operative technique. In addition, most of the patients in Drahush and colleagues'[46] study population underwent minimally invasive lung resections. This combination of maneuvers led to a significantly lower incidence of postoperative prolonged air leak greater than 5 days of 5.7% compared with the national cohort from the Society of Thoracic Surgeons database of 10.9% in similar patients ($P = .0079$).

Miller and colleagues[47] published a larger prospective multicenter case-control trial of 80 patients, 40 of whom underwent staple line reinforcement with bovine pericardium. There was no difference in the duration of postoperative air leak or the number of days of chest tube drainage.

POSTOPERATIVE CHEST TUBE MANAGEMENT

The application of suction compared with water seal for postoperative tube thoracostomy management following pulmonary resection has been studied in multiple randomized trials.[5–8] Efforts at minimizing complications and prolonged hospital stays secondary to air leaks have included the integration of protocol-driven chest tube management into the perioperative care of patients undergoing lung resection.[46]

Early data from Cerfolio and colleagues[6] in 140 consecutive patients in the late 1990s randomized to −20 cm H_2O suction compared with water seal on postoperative day 2 after undergoing elective pulmonary resection. For patients with continued air leaks on suction on postoperative day 3 who were subsequently placed to water seal, all but 1 air leak (7%) resolved postoperative day 4. The investigators noted the importance of quantifying air leaks because leaks graded as 5 to 7 chamber leaks on the Pleura-vac (Sahara Pleura-vac, Deknatel, Boston, MA) were predictive of prolonged postoperative leaks.[6]

Marshall and colleagues[8] subsequently examined 68 patients undergoing elective pulmonary resection including wedge resection, segmental resection, and lobectomy. Patients underwent resection, were briefly kept to suction with −20 cm H_2O intraoperatively, and were randomized to water seal or continued suction starting in the recovery unit. The duration of air leak was shorter in the water-seal cohort (1.5 days) compared with the suction cohort (3.27 days; $P = .05$). In addition, a shorter duration of chest drainage for the water-seal cohort trended toward significance (3.33 days seal vs 5.47 days suction; $P = .06$). However, there were 4 patients in the water-seal group who did undergo crossover to suction with −10 cm H_2O secondary to pneumothoraces greater than or equal to 25% of the hemithorax. All 4 patients were subsequently converted to water seal within 24 hours of being placed to suction.[8]

Brunelli and colleagues[5] conducted a similar study in which patients underwent an elective pulmonary lobectomy for cancer and were randomized to −20 cm H_2O suction or water seal. All patients were initially placed to suction for postoperative day zero and those with an air leak on postoperative day 1 were randomized either to remain on continuous suction or to be placed to water seal. Notably, 80% of the upper lobectomies in this series underwent pleural tenting intraoperatively. There were 72 patients whose chest tubes were placed to water seal and 73 who remained on suction. There was no difference in the rate of prolonged air leak greater than or equal to 7 days (27.8% seal vs 30.1% suction; $P = .8$) or chest tube duration (11.5 days seal vs 10.3 days suction; $P = .2$). Brunelli and colleagues[5] were able to stratify their results by upper versus lower lobectomies; however, results within these groups also did not significantly differ.

SUMMARY

Postoperative PALs following pulmonary resection occur in a substantial portion of patients and place patients at risk for developing postoperative empyema and subsequent interventions. There have been several potential prophylactic maneuvers to prevent PALs; however, no specific technique has emerged as a "silver bullet." Situational circumstances may indicate 1 method of prophylaxis rather than another. For example, upper lobectomies or bilobectomies may lend themselves to pleural tenting, whereas patients undergoing lower lobectomies or bilobectomies may benefit from prophylactic pneumoperitoneum. Furthermore, there have not been any prospective trials in the United States that have examined the use of PGA mesh in a prophylactic or therapeutic setting. In addition, adjunctive measures such as the use of sealants as well as early sealing of chest tubes may provide additional benefit; however, studies that can control for the singular effect of these maneuvers are lacking. The absence of a protocolized or standardized approach to intraoperative pneumostasis and postoperative tube thoracostomy management has led to heterogeneity within the experimental and control arms of published trials.

Current literature has focused on the presence and subsequent resolution of intraoperative air leak. The resolution of intraoperative air leaks in most of the published literature with added procedures for pneumostasis has not led to a consistent improvement in the duration of postoperative air leaks and the prevention of PALs. Therefore, the clinical relevance of intraoperative air leaks is undetermined. Future trials must focus on the definition of a consistent control arm and assess the individual efficacy of each prophylactic measure as well as standardized tube thoracostomy management. Following the assessment of the singular effects of these techniques, focus can be shifted toward combining techniques to maximize efficacy in specific circumstances.

DISCLOSURE

The authors have nothing to disclose.

REFERENCES

1. Liberman M, Muzikansky A, Wright CD, et al. Incidence and risk factors of persistent air leak after major pulmonary resection and use of chemical pleurodesis. Ann Thorac Surg 2010;89:891–8.
2. Mckenna RJ, Fischel RJ, Brenner M, et al. Use of the heimlich valve to shorten hospital stay after lung reduction surgery for emphysema. Ann Thorac Surg 1996;4975:15–7.
3. Dugan KC, Laxmanan B, Murgu S, et al. Incidence of persistent air leaks. Chest 2017;152:417–23.
4. Stolz AJ, Schu J, Lischke R, et al. Predictors of prolonged air leak following pulmonary lobectomy. Eur J Cardiothorac Surg 2005;27:334–6.
5. Brunelli A, Monteverde M, Borri A, et al. Comparison of water seal and suction after pulmonary lobectomy: a prospective, randomized trial. Ann Thorac Surg 2004. https://doi.org/10.1016/j.athoracsur.2003.12.022.
6. Cerfolio RJ, Bass C, Katholi CR. Prospective randomized trial compares suction versus water seal for air leaks. Surg Clin North Am 2001. https://doi.org/10.1016/S0003-4975(01)02474-2.
7. Cerfolio RJ. Advances in thoracostomy tube management. Ann Thorac Surg 2002;82:833–48.
8. Marshall MB, Deeb ME, Bleier JIS, et al. Suction vs water seal after pulmonary resection * a randomized prospective study. Chest 2002;121:831–5.
9. Kawai N, Kawaguchi T, Suzuki S, et al. Low-voltage coagulation, polyglycolic acid sheets, and fibrin glue to control air leaks in lung surgery. Gen Thorac Cardiovasc Surg 2017;65:705–9.
10. Ikeda T, Sasaki M, Yamada N. Controlling air leaks using free pericardial fat pads as surgical sealant in pulmonary resection. Ann Thorac Surg 2015;99:1170–5.
11. Tanaka T, Ueda K, Murakami J. Use of stitching and bioabsorbable mesh and glue to combat prolonged air leaks. Ann Thorac Surg 2018;106:e215–8.
12. Lee S, Park SY, Bae MK, et al. Efficacy of polyglycolic acid sheet after thoracoscopic bullectomy for spontaneous pneumothorax. Ann Thorac Surg 2013;95:1919–23.
13. Saito H, Konno H, Atari M, et al. Management of intersegmental plane on pulmonary segmentectomy concerning postoperative complications. Ann Thorac Surg 2017;103:1773–80.
14. Ueda K, Tanaka T, Jinbo M, et al. Sutureless pneumostasis using polyglycolic acid mesh as artificial pleura during video-assisted major pulmonary resection. Ann Thorac Surg 2007;1858–61.
15. Uramoto H, Takenoyama M. Simple prophylactic fixation for lung torsion. Ann Thorac Surg 2010;90:2028–30.
16. Ueda K, Tanaka T, Hayashi M, et al. Verification of early removal of the chest tube after absorbable

mesh-based pneumostasis subsequent to video-assisted major lung resection for cancer. World J Surg 2012;36:1603–7.

17. Saito T, Kaneda H, Konobu T, et al. The covering with forceps-assisted polymeric biodegradable sheet and endostapling method: a simplified technique for wide coverage and reinforcement of staple-line in video-assisted thoracoscopic bullectomy for spontaneous pneumothorax located on the Wor. Interact Cardiovasc Thorac Surg 2011;103–5. https://doi.org/10.1510/icvts.2010.246124.

18. Okada M, Mimura T, Ikegaki J, et al. A novel video-assisted anatomic segmentectomy technique: Selective segmental inflation via bronchofiberoptic jet followed by cautery cutting. J Thorac Cardiovasc Surg 2007;753–8.

19. Nakamura T, Suzuki K, Mochizuki T, et al. An evaluation of the surgical morbidity of polyglycolic acid felt in pulmonary resections. Surg Today 2010;40:734–7.

20. Maniwa T, Kaneda H, Saito Y, et al. Management of a complicated pulmonary fistula caused by lung cancer using a fibrin glue-soaked polyglycolic acid sheet covered with an intercostal muscle flap located on the World Wide Web at: Management of a complicated pulmonary fistula caused by lung. Interact Cardiovasc Thorac Surg 2009;697–8. https://doi.org/10.1510/icvts.2008.201814.

21. Hirai K, Kawashima T, Takeuchi S, et al. Covering the staple line with a polyglycolic acid sheet after bullectomy for primary spontaneous pneumothorax prevents postoperative recurrent pneumothorax. J Thorac Dis 2015;7:1978–85.

22. Yoshimoto K, Nomori H, Mori T, et al. Comparison of postoperative pulmonary function and air leakage between pleural closure vs. mesh-cover for intersegmental plane in segmentectomy. J Cardiothorac Surg 2011;6:1–6.

23. Ueda K, Tanaka T, Li T, et al. Sutureless pneumostasis using bioabsorbable mesh and glue during major lung resection for cancer: Who are the best candidates? Abbreviations and acronyms. J Thorac Cardiovasc Surg 2010;139:600–5.

24. Venuta F, Diso D, De Giacomo T, et al. Use of a polymeric sealant to reduce air leaks after lobectomy. J Thorac Cardiovasc Surg 2006;2:422–3.

25. Allen MS, Wood DE, Hawkinson RW, et al. Prospective randomized study evaluating a biodegradable polymeric sealant for sealing pulmonary resection. Ann Thorac Surg 2004;77:1792–801.

26. Park BJ, Snider JM, Bates NR, et al. Prospective evaluation of biodegradable polymeric sealant for intraoperative air leaks. J Cardiothorac Surg 2016; 1–8. https://doi.org/10.1186/s13019-016-0563-3.

27. Lequaglie C, Giudice G, Marasco R, et al. Use of a sealant to prevent prolonged air leaks after lung resection: a prospective randomized study. J Cardiothorac Surg 2012;7:1–6.

28. Tan C, Utley M, Paschalides C, et al. A prospective randomized controlled study to assess the effectiveness of CoSeal to seal air leaks in lung surgery. Eur J Cardiothorac Surg 2011;40:304–8.

29. Gologorsky RC, Alabaster AL, Ashiku SK, et al. Progel use is not associated with decreased incidence of postoperative air leak after nonanatomic lung surgery. Perm J 2019;23:8–11.

30. Dango S, Lin R, Hennings E, et al. Initial experience with a synthetic sealant PleuraSeal ™ after pulmonary resections: a prospective study with retrospective case matched controls. J Cardiothorac Surg 2010;5:1–9.

31. D'Andrilli A, Andreetti C, Ibrahim M, et al. A prospective randomized study to assess the efficacy of a surgical sealant to treat air leaks in lung surgery. Eur J Cardiothorac Surg 2009;35:817–21.

32. Moser C, Opitz I, Zhai W, et al. Autologous fibrin sealant reduces the incidence of prolonged air leak and duration of chest tube drainage after lung volume reduction surgery: A prospective randomized blinded study. J Thorac Cardiovasc Surg 2008;843–9. https://doi.org/10.1016/j.jtcvs.2008.02.079.

33. Anegg U, Matzi V, Smolle J, et al. Efficiency of fleece-bound sealing TachoSil) of air leaks in lung surgery: a prospective randomised trial. Eur J Cardiothorac Surg 2007;31:198–202.

34. Filosso PL, Ruf E, Sandri A, et al. Efficacy and safety of human fibrinogen – thrombin patch (TachoSil®) in the treatment of postoperative air leakage in patients submitted to redo surgery for lung malignancies: a randomized trial. Interact Cardiovasc Thorac Surg 2013;16:661–6.

35. Gonfiotti A, Santini PF, Jaus M, et al. Safety and effectiveness of a new fibrin pleural air leak sealant: a multicenter, controlled. Ann Thorac Surg 2011;92: 1217–25.

36. Rena O, Papalia E, Claudio T, et al. Institutional report - Thoracic non-oncologic Air-leak management after upper lobectomy in patients with fused fissure and chronic obstructive pulmonary disease: a pilot trial comparing sealant and standard treatment. Interact Cardiovasc Thorac Surg 2009;9: 973–7.

37. Allama AM. Pleural tent for decreasing air leak following upper lobectomy: a prospective randomised trial. Eur J Cardiothorac Surg 2010;38: 674–8.

38. Uzzaman MM, Robb JD, Mhandu PCE, et al. A meta-analysis assessing the benefits of concomitant pleural tent procedure after upper lobectomy. Ann Thorac Surg 2014;97:365–72.

39. Robinson LA, Preksto D. Pleural tenting during upper lobectomy decreases chest tube time and total hospitalization days. J Thorac Cardiovasc Surg 1997;115:319–27.

40. Okur E, Kir A, Halezeroglu S, et al. Pleural tenting following upper lobectomies or bilobectomies of the lung to prevent residual air space and prolonged air leak. Eur J Cardiothorac Surg 2001;20: 1012–5.

41. Mcconnell PI. Extracellular matrix pleural tent for persistent air leak and air space in a child after upper lobectomy. Ann Thorac Surg 2015;99:321–3.

42. Brunelli A, Al Refai M, Monteverde M, et al. Pleural tent after upper lobectomy: a randomized study of efficacy and duration of effect. Ann Thorac Surg 2002;74:1958–62.

43. Cerfolio RJ, Holman WL, Katholi CR. Pneumoperitoneum after concomitant resection of the right middle and lower lobes (Bilobectomy). Ann Thorac Surg 2000;70:942–7.

44. Okur E, Arisoy Y, Baysungur V, et al. Prophylactic intraoperative pneumoperitoneum decreases pleural space problems after lower lobectomy or bilobectomy of the lung. Thorac Cardiovasc Surg 2009; 160–4. https://doi.org/10.1055/s-2008-1039108.

45. Podgaetz E, Berger J, Small J, et al. Therapeutic pneumoperitoneum: relevant or obsolete in 2015? Thorac Cardiovasc Surg 2017;375–81.

46. Drahush N, Miller AD, Smith JS, et al. Standardized approach to prolonged air leak reduction after pulmonary resection. Ann Thorac Surg 2016;101: 2097–101.

47. Miller JI, Landreneau RJ, Wright CE, et al. A comparative study of buttressed versus nonbuttressed staple line in pulmonary resections. Ann Thorac Surg 2001;71:4975.

48. Takamochi K, Oh S. Prospective randomized trial comparing buttressed versus nonbuttressed stapling in patients undergoing pulmonary lobectomy. Thorac Cardiovasc Surg 2014;696–704.

Surgical Adjuncts During Esophagectomy

Ammara A. Watkins, MD, MPH, Michael S. Kent, MD, Jennifer L. Wilson, MD, MPH*

KEYWORDS

- Esophagectomy complications • Pyloric drainage • Feeding tube • Enteral access
- Anastomotic buttressing • Omentum

KEY POINTS

- During esophagectomy, several intraoperative maneuvers classically thought to mitigate postoperative complications may be indicated.
- Enteral access via jejunostomy tube placement provides reliable enteral nutrition and can prevent malnourishment. Selected patients who exhibit evidence of malnourishment should have enteral access placed before surgery.
- Nasogastric tube decompression at the time of esophagectomy should be used and removed by postoperative day 2 if possible.
- Evidence for pyloric drainage or pyloroplasty is limited. No specific recommendation can be made at this time, but chemical pyloroplasty with botulinum toxin is an option for a temporary pyloric drainage procedure without the long-term side effects associated with pyloromyotomy or surgical pyloroplasty.
- Anastomosis may be buttressed with surrounding tissue. Ideally omentum should be used if available.

INTRODUCTION

Esophagectomy is used for benign and malignant esophageal disease. Although outcomes following esophagectomy have improved over the years, the operation still portends significant morbidity.[1] Herein, the authors critically examine data available for adjunctive surgical procedures, including enteral access, pyloric drainage procedures, nasogastric decompression, and anastomotic buttressing during esophagectomy.

Feeding Tubes

It is common for patients with esophageal cancer to lose up to 15% of their body weight from time of diagnosis to 6 months postoperatively.[3] Randomized clinical trials have shown that early feeding is associated with decreased complications during major gastrointestinal operations.[4–6] There are also some data indicating that length of stay may be shorter and quality of life improved with early feeding.[5,7] Current Enhanced Recovery After Surgery (ERAS) Society guidelines recommend early feeding on days 3 to 6 following esophagectomy.[1] Depending on the patient's clinical status, early feeding may only be possible with tube feeds.

The ERAS Society recommends the use of enteral access via nasoduodenal/nasojejunal tubes (NJ tubes) or jejunostomy feeding tube in patients who are at high risk of malnourishment (**Box 1**).[1] This nutritional assessment should be done at the time of diagnosis or multidisciplinary intervention, ideally with the involvement of a qualified dietitian. Patients should have a feeding tube placed preoperatively or before induction therapy

Division of Thoracic Surgery and Interventional Pulmonology, Beth Israel Deaconess Medical Center, 185 Pilgrim Road, W/D 201, Boston, MA 02215, USA
* Corresponding author.
E-mail address: jwilso10@bidmc.harvard.edu

Thorac Surg Clin 30 (2020) 315–320
https://doi.org/10.1016/j.thorsurg.2020.04.009
1547-4127/20/© 2020 Elsevier Inc. All rights reserved.

Box 1
High-risk indicators for nutritional deficiency[2]

> **Box 1**
> **High-risk indicators for nutritional deficiency[2]**
>
> Severe dysphagia: able to tolerate puree/fluids only
>
> Unintentional weight loss greater than 10%
>
> Body mass index less than 18 kg/m^2
>
> Serum albumin less than 3 g/dL

if there are concerns for malnourishment substantiated by the aforementioned criterion. Interruption of induction therapy for enteral access because of worsening of dysphagia or weight loss should be avoided if possible by preemptively placing feeding tubes in high-risk patients. Intraoperative placement of a feeding tube at time of esophagectomy may have less benefit.[8] The authors favor selective preoperative placement of laparoscopic jejunostomy tubes when needed because jejunostomy tubes are not without their own complications. Although most of these complications are minor, major tube-related complications are associated with morbidity as high as 46% and can require laparotomy in up to 16.7% of patients.[5,8–10]

Other options for enteric access include a nasogastric tube (NG tube), NJ tube, and gastrostomy tube (g-tube; via open or percutaneous technique). A subset of patients may not tolerate preoperative endoscopic placement of a feeding tube and may require operative gastrotomy or jejunostomy placement for reliable enteric access. Feeding tubes traversing the nasopharynx are less comfortable for the patient and have been associated with dislodgement and aspiration.[11] Although rare, there have been some case reports of gastric vasculature compromise following percutaneous gastrotomy (PEG) tube placement.[12] Gastrotomy site metastasis following PEG tube placement has also been reported in individual cases.[13,14] A larger single-center retrospective analysis of patients who underwent gastric tube placement did not find any incidence of these complications.[15] Utilization of the "push" method of PEG placement avoids passing instruments through malignancies and then into healthy tissue, which likely lowers the risk of seeding as compared with the "pull" method of PEG placement.[15] Current National Comprehensive Cancer Network (NCCN) guidelines recommend that gastrotomy placement is more suitable for patients with cervical esophageal cancer who are receiving definitive chemoradiation or for patients with marginally resectable disease.[16] However, data available indicate that g-tube placement, particularly open g-tube or "push" technique PEG placement, is likely a safe alternative for carefully selected patients with resectable esophageal cancer as an alternative to jejunostomy tube or NG-/NJ-tube placement.

Nasogastric Decompression

ERAS Society guidelines strongly recommend intraoperative NG tube placement for postoperative decompression with the caveat that early removal (postoperative day 2) be pursued when appropriate.[1] Two randomized control trials have assessed the use of postoperative NG tube decompression.[17,18] Shackcloth and colleagues[17] compared standard NG tube decompression with early removal (on postoperative day 2) versus no NG tube decompression. Higher pulmonary complications were seen in the group without NG tube decompression.[17] Mistry and colleagues[18] compared early (postoperative day 2) versus delayed NG tube removal and found no difference in pulmonary or other complications. As expected, patients had less pain complaints about the NG tube when it was removed early. However, the group with early NG tube removal had higher reinsertion rates as compared with the group that underwent delayed removal.[18] A recent metaanalysis confirmed early removal of NG tubes is not associated with increased rates of anastomotic leak, pulmonary complications, or mortality. Notably, this study also found no difference in pulmonary or anastomotic complications whether nasogastric decompression was omitted, although analysis included retrospective data.[11]

Pyloric Drainage Procedures

Delayed gastric emptying occurs in up to 50% of patients following esophagectomy because of the truncal vagotomy that is part of resection, tubularization of the stomach, and gastric pull-up.[3,19] It is impossible to determine which patients will develop gastric outlet obstruction and benefit from pyloric drainage. Four options exist to address this problem at the time of surgery: no intervention, pyloroplasty, pyloromyotomy, or chemical pyloroplasty. Although pyloromyotomy and pyloroplasty were historically well accepted, there is now considerable debate about their efficacy.[20] Advocates of the drainage procedures cite the low morbidity and potential to minimize postoperative conduit dilation, which may lead to anastomotic leak. Those critical of these interventions espouse the long-term benefits of an intact pylorus. In addition, delayed gastric outlet obstruction has been shown to be effectively treated with endoscopic measures, including

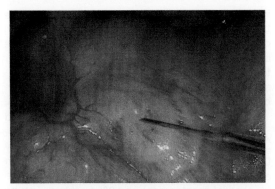

Fig. 1. Botulinum toxin injection into pylorus.

balloon dilation, botulinum toxin injection, and endoscopic per-oral pyloromyotomy.[21]

In summary, the data surrounding pyloric drainage procedures are mixed and limited. There are insufficient data to recommend drainage procedures over not performing pyloric drainage. Several retrospective series have found no difference in rates of delayed gastric outlet obstruction after pyloromyotomy or pyloroplasty.[22–24] A prospective study of 242 patients undergoing

esophagectomy with a gastric conduit found no difference in rates of gastric outlet obstruction among patients who did and did not receive a pyloromyotomy.[25] In contrast, a metaanalysis of 9 trials and 553 esophagectomy patients randomized to pyloromyotomy versus no pyloric drainage procedure found a lower risk of gastric outlet obstruction for patients treated with pyloromyotomy (odds ratio: 0.18, 95% confidence interval [CI]: 0.03–0.97, $P<.046$).[26] However, this metaanalysis found no difference in operative mortality, anastomotic leaks, or pulmonary complications.[26] A more recent systematic review did find nonstatistically significant trends toward decreased gastric outlet obstruction and lower anastomotic leaks.[27]

Given the inconclusive data available, current ERAS guidelines do not make a recommendation on the role of pyloric drainage.[1] The authors selectively use chemical pyloroplasty with 200 units of botulinum toxin injected on the anterior surface of the pylorus (**Fig. 1**); this can alternatively be done in 4 quadrants. Although expensive, botulinum chemical pyloroplasty is a simple, safe, and temporary gastric outlet procedure that provides

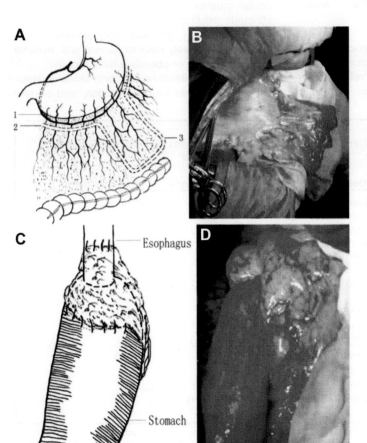

Fig. 2. Technique for omental flap construction. (*A*) Technique for harvesting the omental graft: (*1*) right gastroepiploic artery; (*2*) mobilized site of omentum for harvesting the pedicle omental flap; (*3*) pedicle omental flap. (*B*) Harvesting a pedicle omental flap during an operation. (*C*) The method for wrapping of the pedicle omental flap around the esophagogastric anastomotic site after esophagectomy. (*D*) Wrapping of the pedicle omental flap around the esophagogastric anastomotic site after esophagectomy during an operation. (*From* Dai et al. with permission.[33])

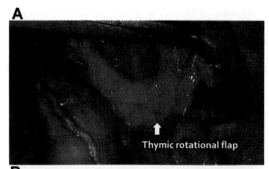

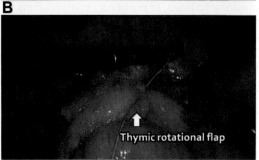

Fig. 3. Thymic rotational flap. (*A*) Fully mobilized thymic rotational flap elevated by instrument. Esophageal anastomosis staple line is visible. (*B*) Circumferential tension-free rotational flap around esophageal anastomosis.

the early benefit of a gastric outlet procedure and avoids long-term complications, including biliary reflux and dumping syndrome.[28] In 1 retrospective analysis, however, intraoperative botulinum injection was associated with more acid reflux than pyloromyotomy and pyloroplasty at the time of 6-month follow-up.[29] If chemical pyloroplasty is inadequate in the long term with recurrent symptoms of delayed gastric emptying, then endoscopic or laparoscopic drainage procedures may be offered to the patient.

Anastomotic Buttressing

Despite improvements in surgical techniques, esophageal leak rates remain significant at 12% for cervical anastomoses and 9% for intrathoracic anastomoses.[30] Buttress of an intrathoracic anastomosis using a pedicled omental flap has demonstrated decreased leak and stricture rates in large retrospective series and 2 prospective randomized control trials.[31–34] Typically, the omental pedicle is created by preserving 2 to 4 perforating arteries from the right gastroepiploic artery (**Fig. 2**),[33] and this is transposed into the chest and wrapped around the anastomosis medial to lateral like a scarf. The omentum pedicle surrounds the entire anastomosis and lies along the gastric conduit lesser curvature staple line. Intercostal muscle or thymus may also be used, although existing published data are limited to the use in airway and pulmonary operations.[35,36] Thymus is relatively easy to harvest with minimal added morbidity or operative time (**Fig. 3**).

Although the literature supports omental wrapping, it is not yet routine practice, and current

Table 1
Summary of Enhanced Recovery After Surgery Society recommendations for operative adjuncts to esophagectomy

Element	Recommendation	Level of Evidence	Recommendation Grade
Enteric feeding tube	Early enteral feeding should be used. If a patient is high risk for malnutrition, a feeding tube should be placed preoperatively. Feeding jejunostomy or NG/NJ tubes are preferred	Moderate	Moderate
Nasogastric decompression	Should be used postoperatively but with early discontinuation (postoperative day 2)	Moderate	Strong
Pyloric drainage procedure	No specific recommendation can be made given the limited data available	Low	Strong
Anastomotic buttress	Not addressed in ERAS Society recommendations		

Adapted from Low DE, Alderson D, Cecconello I, et al. International consensus on standardization of data collection for complications associated with esophagectomy: Esophagectomy Complications Consensus Group (ECCG). Ann Surg 2015;262:286–94; with permission.

ERAS guidelines do not include any discussion on anastomotic buttressing.[1,35,37] Arguments against routine omental wrapping include potential obstruction at the diaphragm by the omentum and omental bleeding secondary to traction. In addition, a wrap may contribute to a complex phlegmon should there be an anastomotic leak, potentially complicating the leak management. In fact, the authors' group selectively used a thymic rotational flap to buttress the anastomosis for minimally invasive Ivor-Lewis esophagectomy until they encountered a complex postoperative leak with a large phlegmon component that was difficult to manage. Nevertheless, omental wrapping may be a useful addition, not a substitution, to a well-perfused conduit and technically optimized anastomosis. Surgeons may consider adding the buttress to their esophagectomy technique.

SUMMARY

Esophagectomy is a complex operation fraught with numerous potential complications. **Table 1** summarizes available adjuncts to surgery and their ERAS Society recommendations with level of evidence. In sum, enteral access should be pursued preoperatively for patients at high risk for malnutrition. NG tube drainage should be used with the caveat of early discontinuation when feasible. All available pyloric drainage procedures have mixed and limited data; these maneuvers should be used selectively. Although not addressed by the ERAS Society, anastomotic buttressing with omentum should be considered because data indicate it may reduce the incidence and severity of anastomotic leaks.

DISCLOSURE

The authors have no disclosures or conflicts of interest to report.

REFERENCES

1. Low DE, Allum W, De Manzoni G, et al. Guidelines for perioperative care in esophagectomy: Enhanced Recovery After Surgery (ERAS((R))) Society recommendations. World J Surg 2019;43:299–330.
2. Low DE, Alderson D, Cecconello I, et al. International consensus on standardization of data collection for complications associated with esophagectomy: Esophagectomy Complications Consensus Group (ECCG). Ann Surg 2015;262:286–94.
3. Donington JS. Functional conduit disorders after esophagectomy. Thorac Surg Clin 2006;16:53–62.
4. Knight AW, Blackmon SH. The ongoing debate regarding optimal nutritional routes following esophagectomy. J Thorac Dis 2016;8:3006–8.
5. Al-Temimi MH, Dyurgerova AM, Kidon M, et al. Feeding jejunostomy tube placed during esophagectomy: is there an effect on postoperative outcomes? Perm J 2019;23.
6. Zheng R, Devin CL, Pucci MJ, et al. Optimal timing and route of nutritional support after esophagectomy: a review of the literature. World J Gastroenterol 2019;25:4427–36.
7. Sun HB, Li Y, Liu XB, et al. Early oral feeding following McKeown minimally invasive esophagectomy: an open-label, randomized, controlled, noninferiority trial. Ann Surg 2018;267:435–42.
8. Alvarez-Sarrado E, Mingol Navarro F, J Rosellón R, et al. Feeding jejunostomy after esophagectomy cannot be routinely recommended. Analysis of nutritional benefits and catheter-related complications. Am J Surg 2019;217:114–20.
9. Weijs TJ, Berkelmans GH, Nieuwenhuijzen GA, et al. Routes for early enteral nutrition after esophagectomy. A systematic review. Clin Nutr 2015;34:1–6.
10. Berkelmans GHK, Fransen L, Weijs TJ, et al. The long-term effects of early oral feeding following minimal invasive esophagectomy. Dis Esophagus 2018; 31:1–8.
11. Weijs TJ, Kumagai K, Berkelmans GH, et al. Nasogastric decompression following esophagectomy: a systematic literature review and meta-analysis. Dis Esophagus 2017;30:1–8.
12. Ohnmacht GA, Allen MS, Cassivi SD, et al. Percutaneous endoscopic gastrostomy risks rendering the gastric conduit unusable for esophagectomy. Dis Esophagus 2006;19:311–2.
13. Becker G, Hess CF, Grund KE, et al. Abdominal wall metastasis following percutaneous endoscopic gastrostomy. Support Care Cancer 1995;3:313–6.
14. Stockeld D, Fagerberg J, Granstrom L, et al. Percutaneous endoscopic gastrostomy for nutrition in patients with oesophageal cancer. Eur J Surg 2001; 167:839–44.
15. Saeed SM, Fontaine JP, Dam AN, et al. Is preoperative G-tube use safe for esophageal cancer patients? J Am Coll Nutr 2019;1–6. https://doi.org/10.1080/07315724.2019.1646168.
16. Esophageal and esophagogastric cancers (version 1.2020). Available at: https://www.nccn.org/professionals/physician_gls/pdf/esophageal.pdf. Accessed April 11, 2020.
17. Shackcloth MJ, McCarron E, Kendall J, et al. Randomized clinical trial to determine the effect of nasogastric drainage on tracheal acid aspiration following oesophagectomy. Br J Surg 2006;93: 547–52.
18. Mistry RC, Vijayabhaskar R, Karimundackal G, et al. Effect of short-term vs prolonged nasogastric decompression on major postesophagectomy complications: a parallel-group, randomized trial. Arch Surg 2012;147:747–51.

19. Konradsson M, Nilsson M. Delayed emptying of the gastric conduit after esophagectomy. J Thorac Dis 2019;11:S835–44.

20. Gaur P, Swanson SJ. Should we continue to drain the pylorus in patients undergoing an esophagectomy? Dis Esophagus 2014;27:568–73.

21. Zhang L, Hou SC, Miao JB, et al. Risk factors for delayed gastric emptying in patients undergoing esophagectomy without pyloric drainage. J Surg Res 2017;213:46–50.

22. Fritz S, Feilhauer K, Schaudt A, et al. Pylorus drainage procedures in thoracoabdominal esophagectomy–a single-center experience and review of the literature. BMC Surg 2018;18:13.

23. Palmes D, Weilinghoff M, Colombo-Benkmann M, et al. Effect of pyloric drainage procedures on gastric passage and bile reflux after esophagectomy with gastric conduit reconstruction. Langenbecks Arch Surg 2007;392:135–41.

24. Velanovich V. Esophagogastrectomy without pyloroplasty. Dis Esophagus 2003;16:243–5.

25. Lanuti M, de Delva PE, Wright CD, et al. Post-esophagectomy gastric outlet obstruction: role of pyloromyotomy and management with endoscopic pyloric dilatation. Eur J Cardiothorac Surg 2007;31:149–53.

26. Urschel JD, Blewett CJ, Young JE, et al. Pyloric drainage (pyloroplasty) or no drainage in gastric reconstruction after esophagectomy: a meta-analysis of randomized controlled trials. Dig Surg 2002;19:160–4.

27. Arya S, Markar SR, Karthikesalingam A, et al. The impact of pyloric drainage on clinical outcome following esophagectomy: a systematic review. Dis Esophagus 2015;28:326–35.

28. Martin JT, Federico JA, McKelvey AA, et al. Prevention of delayed gastric emptying after esophagectomy: a single center's experience with botulinum toxin. Ann Thorac Surg 2009;87:1708–13 [discussion: 13–4].

29. Eldaif SM, Lee R, Adams KN, et al. Intrapyloric botulinum injection increases postoperative esophagectomy complications. Ann Thorac Surg 2014;97:1959–64 [discussion: 64–5].

30. Kassis ES, Kosinski AS, Ross P Jr, et al. Predictors of anastomotic leak after esophagectomy: an analysis of the society of thoracic surgeons general thoracic database. Ann Thorac Surg 2013;96:1919–26.

31. Sepesi B, Swisher SG, Walsh GL, et al. Omental reinforcement of the thoracic esophagogastric anastomosis: an analysis of leak and reintervention rates in patients undergoing planned and salvage esophagectomy. J Thorac Cardiovasc Surg 2012;144:1146–50.

32. Bhat MA, Dar MA, Lone GN, et al. Use of pedicled omentum in esophagogastric anastomosis for prevention of anastomotic leak. Ann Thorac Surg 2006;82:1857–62.

33. Dai JG, Zhang ZY, Min JX, et al. Wrapping of the omental pedicle flap around esophagogastric anastomosis after esophagectomy for esophageal cancer. Surgery 2011;149:404–10.

34. Yuan Y, Hu Y, Xie TP, et al. Omentoplasty for preventing anastomotic leaks after esophagogastrostomy. Surgery 2011;149:853–4.

35. Bertheuil N, Cusumano C, Meal C, et al. Skin perforator flap pedicled by intercostal muscle for repair of a tracheobronchoesophageal fistula. Ann Thorac Surg 2017;103:e571–3.

36. Wurtz A, Juthier F, Conti M, et al. The "thymopericardial fat flap": a versatile flap in thoracic and cardiovascular surgery. J Thorac Cardiovasc Surg 2011;141:841–2, 842.e1.

37. Fukumoto Y, Matsunaga T, Shishido Y, et al. Successful repair using thymus pedicle flap for tracheoesophageal fistula: a case report. Surg Case Rep 2018;4:49.

Interventional Pulmonology
A Brave New World

Hardeep S. Kalsi, MBBs, IBSc[a], Ricky Thakrar, MBBs, PhD, IBSc[a],
Andre F. Gosling, MD[b], Shahzad Shaefi, MD, MPH[b,1],
Neal Navani, MD, MSc, PhD[a,*,1]

KEYWORDS

• Bronchoscopy • Interventional pulmonology • Lung cancer

KEY POINTS

- Interventional pulmonology has evolved into a major field with a crucial role in patient care pathways.
- Implementation of lung cancer screening has meant that more patients with peripheral lung nodules are detected and has increased the need for advanced and innovative bronchoscopic approaches.
- Bronchoscopic intervention commonly is used to treat benign and malignant airway obstruction in order to improve symptoms and performance status, which may allow access to further therapies previously considered not appropriate.
- There are several newer diagnostic and therapeutic bronchoscopic approaches now available in clinical practice and this review aims to provide a more detailed insight in to their utility.

INTRODUCTION

The past decade has seen somewhat of a shift away from diagnostic thoracic surgery due largely to a rapid development in technologies in interventional pulmonology (IP). Multidisciplinary thoracic cancer diagnosis and treatment involving IP, thoracic surgery, and oncology are increasingly adopted approaches. Increased focus on lung cancer screening and early detection, in particular, to aid diagnosis of peripheral pulmonary lesions (PPLs) has meant that the incidence of detection is likely to rise. Determining etiology is essential, because lesions between 0.8 cm and 2 cm have an 18% prevalence of malignancy, whereas those above 2 cm have a risk that climbs to 50%.[1,2] Therefore, timely and accurate location, sampling, and diagnosis of PPL through a minimally invasive, less morbid approach increasingly are vital.

Computed tomography (CT)-guided biopsy often is performed to investigate PPLs but suffers somewhat from certain limitations. Anatomic accessibility, size of lesion (<10 mm associated with lower diagnostic yield), and patient comorbidities all play a role in candidacy. This technique also carries a risk of pneumothorax, reported overall at approximately 15% to 20% but with a heterogeneous risk profile as high as 60% in biopsies of lesions under 20 mm.[3,4]

Surgical biopsy still has a role to play, although this has diminished over the past decade.[5] The main advantage remains conferring high diagnostic yield but with higher perioperative risk stratification than IP techniques. Mediastinoscopy anatomically is disadvantaged due to reduced ability to access posteriorly located subcarinal nodes and lower hilar stations (11R & 11L).

[a] Division of Medicine, Lungs for Living Research Centre, UCL Respiratory, University College London, Rayne Building, 5 University Street, London, UK; [b] Department of Anesthesia, Critical Care and Pain Medicine, Beth Israel Deaconess Medical Center, 1 Deaconess Road, Boston, MA, USA
[1] Co-senior authors.
* Corresponding author.
E-mail address: n.navani@ucl.ac.uk

Thorac Surg Clin 30 (2020) 321–338
https://doi.org/10.1016/j.thorsurg.2020.04.001
1547-4127/20/© 2020 Elsevier Inc. All rights reserved.

Additionally, proceeding straight to surgery in PPLs is not straightforward either because it has been demonstrated that lobectomy without prior histologic confirmation of malignancy is associated with benign pathology in up to a third of cases.[6–8] This review, therefore, focuses on current indications and techniques for advanced diagnostic and therapeutic bronchoscopy available in concert with traditional thoracic surgery in the management of benign and malignant thoracic disease.

ADVANCED DIAGNOSTIC BRONCHOSCOPY
Convex Endobronchial Ultrasound

Endobronchial ultrasound (EBUS) and transbronchial needle aspiration (TBNA) revolutionized the approach to lung cancer staging and diagnosis of mediastinal disease. Use of a convex linear ultrasound array positioned at the distal end of a flexible bronchoscope allows visualization of mediastinal lymph structures outside of the airway and real-time sampling (**Fig. 1**). This technique is associated with a high sensitivity, with tissue acquisition shown to be sufficient for immunohistochemistry and molecular analysis for targetable mutations.[9]

Prior to the advent of EBUS, staging of disease was based on CT, PET imaging, and surgical sampling. CT imaging alone, however, has a sensitivity of 55% for detecting mediastinal lymph node metastasis, and 40% of CT-diagnosed lymph nodes considered malignant are actually benign whereas conversely, 20% of those under 10 mm are proved metastatic.[10,11] Fluorodeoxyglucose (FDG)-PET improves on this and currently is the gold standard for detection of extrapulmonary metastases. While conferring 85% sensitivity for mediastinal lymph node metastasis, it does carry a poor specificity for large mediastinal lymph nodes[12,13]; 20% of enlarged FDG-avid lymph nodes are attributable to nonmalignant disease.

The landmark multicenter randomized ASTER trial compared surgical staging to EBUS/endoscopic ultrasound followed by surgical staging.[14] The trial demonstrated greater sensitivity for mediastinal nodal metastases (94% in the EBUS/endoscopic ultrasound group vs 77% in the surgical group) and fewer unnecessary thoracotomies. In another study, compared with mediastinoscopy alone, diagnostic accuracy using EBUS was superior, 91% versus 78%.[15] It must be acknowledged that this may well be in part be due to nonaccessible posteriorly located subcarinal lymph nodes via mediastinoscopy rather than overall decreased accuracy. Furthermore, there has been an effect on timing of progression through patient care pathways to treatment with EBUS. In a UK trial of 133 patients with stages I–IIIa disease, median time to treatment was shorter in those who underwent EBUS-TBNA instead of conventional diagnosis and staging, 14 days versus 29 days, respectively, with a post hoc analysis showing an increase in median survival in non–small cell lung cancer (NSCLC) patients who underwent EBUS (**Fig. 2**).[16]

Peripheral Pulmonary Lesions

Fluoroscopy
Fluoroscopic imaging during bronchoscopy may adjunctively improve the diagnostic yield when targeting PPLs (**Fig. 3**). In a meta-analysis of 18 studies encompassing 1687 patients, use of fluoroscopy with bronchoscopy was associated with a 60% diagnostic success rate versus 45% when carried out via bronchoscopy alone.[17] The presence of a bronchus leading directly to a PPL on CT scan, on-site pathology assessment, and lesion size greater than 3 cm were associated with a higher diagnostic yield.

Cone-beam computed tomography
The cone beam-CT (CBCT) method involves the use of an x-ray C-arm scanner, which rotates in

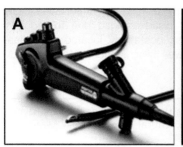
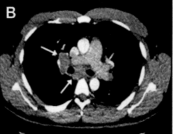
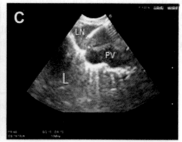

Fig. 1. EBUS-TBNA. (*A*) EBUS bronchoscope with convex ultrasound array at tip. (*B*) CT chest demonstrating hilar and mediastinal lymphadenopathy in a 28-year-old patient with systemic weight loss and fatigue. (*C*) Ultrasound image at bronchoscopy showing EBUS needle in hilar lymph node (LN), adjacent pulmonary vessel (PV), and lung (L) with pleural enhancement and comet tail appearance. (*Courtesy of* Pentax Medical, Tokyo, Japan.)

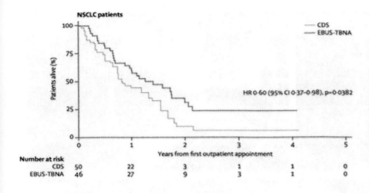

Fig. 2. Survival outcomes in NSCLC patients who underwent conventional staging and diagnosis versus EBUS-TBNA staging. (*From* Navani N, Nankivell M, Lawrence DR, et al. Lung cancer diagnosis and staging with endobronchial ultrasound-guided transbronchial needle aspiration compared with conventional approaches: an open-label, pragmatic, randomised controlled trial. Lancet Respir Med. 2015;3(4):287; with permission.)

real time during the procedure around a patient to produce a CT image. Although the image quality is not that of a diagnostic CT, it is sufficient to allow identification of a PPL and bronchoscopic equipment aimed at targeting this.[18] CBCT in conjunction with other approaches has been shown effective, with a reported diagnostic yield of up to 84% in diagnosing PPLs.[19]

Radial endobronchial ultrasound
The radial EBUS technique consists of a flexible catheter with an oscillating ultrasound probe at its tip, providing a 360o assessment of a distal airway. This may be effective particularly in PPLs where a bronchus sign is present (see **Fig. 3**).[20–22] Reported diagnostic yields range from 58% to 88% in the literature. One meta-analysis reviewed 16 studies involving 1420 patients undergoing radial EBUS-guided bronchoscopy for investigation of a PPL. The sensitivity rate for detection was 0.73 (0.70–0.76).[23] A subsequent larger meta-analysis of 57 different studies and 7872 PPLs found a diagnostic yield rate of 70.6%, with the presence of malignancy, bronchus sign, or lesion greater than 2 cm associated

with a higher success rate.[24] The presence of the probe within a lesion rather than adjacent to it also was more favorable.

Electromagnetic navigational bronchoscopy
Distal targeting of a PPL with a bronchus sign can be limited by inaccessibility due to the physical dimensions of a bronchoscope. Electromagnetic navigational bronchoscopy is a method that can be used to overcome this to diagnose lesions, sample lymph nodes, site treatment catheters (eg, radiotherapy), and place fiducial markers to assist prospective surgery.[25] Prebronchoscopy planning CT and virtual reconstruction can be synchronized with live bronchoscopy to provide navigation (**Fig. 4**). An electromagnetic plate beneath the plate permits a smaller steerable working channel to be advanced from the bronchoscope once the latter's limitations are reached to distally access a lesion. The NAVIGATE study demonstrated electromagnetic navigational bronchoscopy is a safe and effective modality in diagnosing PPLs (radial-EBUS assisted in some cases), and to help site fiducial markers for surgery or stereotactic radiotherapy.[26,27]

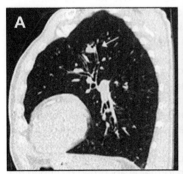
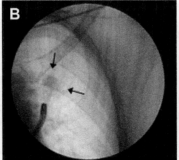
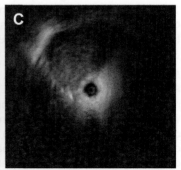

Fig. 3. Fluoroscopy and radial EBUS. (*A*) Left upper lesion with bronchus sign in a renal transplant patient on immunosuppression. (*B*) Bronchoscopy with fluoroscopy to help target the lesion and subsegmental airway. (*C*) Ultrasound image obtained on radial EBUS showing lesion between the 10-o'clock and 1-o'clock positions.

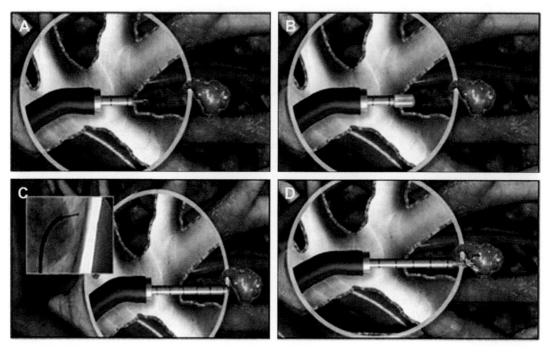

Fig. 4. Bronchoscopic transparenchymal nodule access (BTPNA). (*A*) Initial puncture through a predetermined target in an airway wall. (*B*) Dilatation of the access point to establish the beginning of a tract. (*C*) Careful tunneling creating a tract toward the target parenchymal lesion. (*D*) Biopsy and sampling of peripheral parenchymal lesion. (*Courtesy of* Broncus Medical Inc., San Jose, CA.)

Bronchoscopic transparenchymal nodule access

The novel approach, bronchoscopic transparenchymal nodule access, employs augmented fluoroscopy after preprocedural planning of a path toward a peripheral parenchymal lesion through an airway wall. It does not rely on the need for a bronchus sign because the procedure involves puncturing an airway wall, dilation, and passage of a catheter through a tract toward a lesion and subsequently sampling to be performed (**Fig. 5**). A pilot human study in 12 patients demonstrated adequate diagnostic sampling was achieved in 83% of cases.[28] A further small study of 6 patients demonstrated a malignancy diagnosis rate of 100% in the 5 individuals able to undergo the procedure.[29] A multicenter trial across 9 sites aiming to recruit 200 patients currently is under way.

Robotic bronchoscopy

Robotic bronchoscopy represents potentially the most advanced future platform on the horizon, with the possibility of a thinner, more flexible bronchoscope potentially being able to navigate more distally throughout the bronchial tree to interrogate disease.[30,31] A small feasibility and safety study assessing its use in investigation of pulmonary lesions in a 15-patient cohort successfully was reported without adverse events encountered.[32]

Autofluorescence bronchoscopy

Autofluorescence bronchoscopy (AFB) can be used to detect preinvasive malignant disease by utilizing the differences between red light and green light absorption demonstrated by abnormal and normal epithelium.[33–35] In abnormal mucosa, there is an increase in fluorophores, which absorb and emit fluorescence when irradiated with light (see **Fig. 5**).[36] It is associated with a 1.4-fold to 6.3-fold increase in sensitivity in detecting preinvasive disease compared with white light alone, and a meta-analysis showed a pooled sensitivity of 85% for white light bronchoscopy (WLB) combined with AFB versus 43% for WLB alone.[37] A key aspect to consider, however, is that AFB has a lower specificity than WLB because nonspecific airway changes often also can lead to abnormal fluorescence.[38]

Narrow band imaging (NBI) demonstrates similar advantages and is helpful in detecting changes, such as vessel growth, tortuosity, and microvascular patterns associated with angiogenesis, which develop during early phases of premalignant disease (see **Fig. 5**).[39,40] This is achieved through emission of blue light and green light bandwidths. The former is absorbed by superficial capillaries in the mucosa and the latter by submucosal blood vessels. The combined effect allows

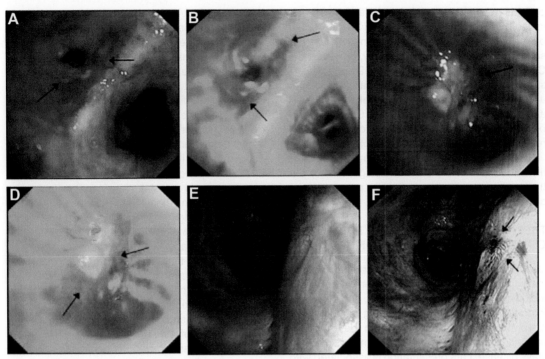

Fig. 5. Autofluorescence imaging (AFI) and NBI. (*A, B*) Mucosal abnormality (*arrow*) in superior lingula on white light and abnormal fluorescence; biopsies confirming carcinoma in-situ recurrence. (*C, D*) New apical left lower lobe lesion in the same patient with corresponding abnormal fluorescence; biopsy demonstrated severely dysplastic epithelium and surgical resection confirmed a new invasive squamous cell carcinoma. (*E*) Left main bronchus mucosa under light bronchoscopy after previous laser therapy for endobronchial carcinoid. (*F*) Appearances under NBI, which show cluster of microvessels; biopsy confirming residual carcinoid disease.

more detailed assessment of the mucosa for signs of angiogenesis, which may accompany premalignant changes or early invasive disease.[40–42] In 1 meta-analysis of 6 studies, NBI demonstrated improved sensitivity compared with WLB (86% vs 70%) and specificity (81% vs 66%) in detecting early premalignant or invasive airway disease.[43]

Both modalities can prove effective in screening for disease recurrence in cases of previous carcinoma in situ at a surgical margin or in individuals with previously proved dysplastic airway lesions (eg, smokers), which may evolve over time. They also can be used to assess for response to treatment after previous direct endobronchial management, such as debulking and laser therapy.

Transbronchial lung cryobiopsy

Transbronchial lung biopsies have long been hindered by small tissue acquisition and crush artifact distorting analysis. Use of a flexible cryotherapy catheter probe inserted through a bronchoscope to obtain larger transbronchial lung cryobiopsies (TBLCBs) has shown increasing promise.[44] Acquired tissue samples are larger (5–10 mm), with architecture maintained without distortion,

allowing more accurate analysis.[45] Surgical lung biopsies (SLBs), although conferring high diagnostic rates, are associated with a 30-day mortality rate of 2% in cases of video-assisted thoracoscopic biopsies and 43% in open lung biopsies.[46] TBLCB also can be performed as a day-case procedure under monitored anesthesia care, thereby reducing risk and minimizing hospital inpatient stay. The main risks are pneumothorax (12%) and significant airway bleeding (39%), the latter managed through use of an endobronchial balloon blocker at sampling to occlude a segmental airway temporarily.[47]

Ravaglia and colleagues[48] compared 150 patients who underwent SLB versus 297 who underwent TBLCB. Mortality rates and length of admission were higher in surgical patients, with diagnostic yield rates of 99% (SLB) and 82.8% (TBLCB). A retrospective review of 117 patients with undiagnosed interstitial lung disease compared outcomes in 58 who underwent TBLCB versus 59 who had SLB. Diagnostic confidence was similar in both groups, at 63% in the TBLCB group and 65% in the SLB group.[49] Contrastingly, a prospective 2-center analysis in 2019 of 21 patients who underwent sequential TBLCB followed by SLB of the same anatomic region noted only a 48% concordance in diagnosis between sampling methods.[50] More recently, however, the COLDICE study, carried out across 9 tertiary interstitial lung disease centers in Australia, pointed to a 70.8% diagnostic agreement between TBLCB and SLB, with this as high as 95% in high-probability/definite diagnosis cases when reviewed by a specialist multidisciplinary team.[51]

TBLCB has a lower risk profile than surgical profile but its role in the diagnostic algorithm of patients with interstitial lung disease remains to be clarified.

THERAPEUTIC BRONCHOSCOPY FOR CENTRAL AIRWAY OBSTRUCTION

Central airway obstruction (CAO) is defined specifically as obstruction of the central airways, including the trachea, main bronchi, and bronchus intermedius. Symptoms, including cough, dyspnea, wheeze, and stridor, often develop late and may be misdiagnosed as asthma or small airways disease. Late presentation is associated with high morbidity and mortality; hence, clinician awareness is key to prevent potential respiratory failure and asphyxia. Prompt clinical assessment, peak flow measurement (as an indicator of proximal airway airflow), and cross-sectional imaging are paramount to enabling rapid diagnosis and guide management, which often manifests as emergency rescue measures.

CAO can be classified as malignant, in the context of cancer, or as benign/nonmalignant, for example, stricture secondary to vasculitis. A majority of cases are due to primary lung carcinoma, where approximately 20% of patients develop clinically significant CAO. Squamous cell carcinomas account for most of these, but rarer forms, such as adenocystic carcinomas, which classically can affect the central airways, should be noted. The types of CAO are outlined in **Fig. 6**. An additional factor to consider when assessing CAO is the presence of viable lower airways and distal lung, which may influence whether intervention is appropriate.

Laser Photoresection

Laser ablation is an important tool in the management of CAO, most importantly endoluminal disease. It can be used to vaporize, coagulate, devascularize, and debulk airway lesions. In benign disease, a laser also can be used in conjunction with balloon dilatation therapy to treat strictures by cutting superficial fibrotic airway bands. The effects of laser therapy are more immediate and, therefore, can be very helpful in the context of palliative disease control and symptom relief. There are several types of lasers, each with different characteristics that in turn may guide their role (**Table 1**); however, Nd:YAG often is the type used most commonly in bronchoscopy.[52]

Bronchoscopic application can be performed through flexible or rigid bronchoscopy and is done best under general anesthesia. Given the potential depth penetration, it is important that application ensures it is fired toward the airway lumen and not perpendicular to the wall (**Fig. 7**). Protective eyewear is mandatory to avoid retinal injury to operators and health care professionals. The most concerning risk is endobronchial fire, with a Fio_2 below 40% strictly advised in all cases when delivering therapy within the bronchial tree.[53] Short efficient time usage is important for this reason and often improves with operator experience. Other complications include bleeding, airway perforation, pneumothorax, hemorrhage, infection, and fistula formation.

Data on use of laser therapy often are retrospective and not randomized or controlled. Furthermore, it often is used in a multimodality approach with other therapies at the time of bronchoscopy. In 1 study comparing Nd:YAG laser therapy in conjunction with external beam radiotherapy versus control (external beam radiotherapy alone), it was seen that use of additional laser therapy improved survival.[54] A case series assessing laser therapy alone, brachytherapy alone, and both together observed a longer median survival time in the combined cohort, 264 days, versus 111 days and 115 days, respectively.[55] Laser therapy also has been shown effective in treating endobronchial carcinoid disease, negating the need for invasive surgery.[56–58]

Argon Plasma Photocoagulation

Argon plasma photocoagulation (APC) first was described in the treatment of gastrointestinal bleeding in 1981 and subsequently has been expanded in its uses to various settings.[59] It uses nonionized argon gas to which a voltage electrical current is applied once it is injected on to a target area. This leads to ionization of the argon gas, generating a monopolar current in the target tissue and subsequent heat generation.[60,61] Its small-depth penetration means it is best suited for treatment of superficial disease and is effective in achieving hemostasis at mucosal surfaces. Due to the movement of the argon gas around bends, it can be effective to treat disease bifurcation points or distal locations within the bronchial tree. The risks related to APC are similar to those

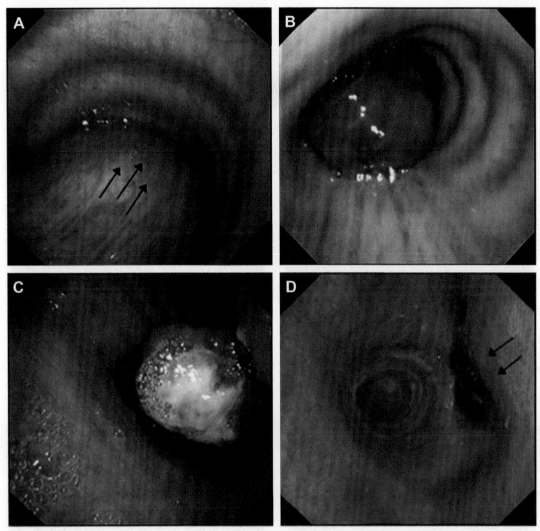

Fig. 6. Types of CAO. (*A*) Extrinsic compression due to malignant disease outside of the trachea (posteriorly in this case). (*B*) Intraluminal obstruction secondary to a tracheal tumor within the airway lumen. (*C, D*) Mixed obstruction, best seen postdebulking (cryoextraction and laser) with endoluminal tumor and left tracheal wall extrinsic compression.

Table 1
Types of lasers and their respective properties

Laser	Wavelength, nm	Penetration Depth	Vaporization	Coagulation	Cutting
APC	516	1–2 mm	–	++	+
KTP	532	0.8 mm	++	++	+
Diode	808	8–10 mm	+	++	+++
Nd:YAG	1060	4–6 mm	+++	+++	+
Thulium	1940	0.4 mm	++	++	+++
CO_2	10,600	0.3 mm	+	–	+++

Plus and minus symbols refer to level of activity where -, refers to no activity and +++, refers to significant activity.

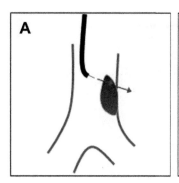 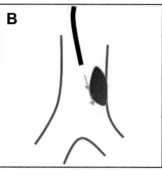

Fig. 7. Endobronchial laser therapy. (*A*) Incorrect positioning of laser, raising risk of airway perforation through airway wall. (*B*) Correct laser application with beam firing at lesion but in direction of airway lumen distally.

of laser photoresection; Laser therapy has also been shown to be effective in treating endobronchial disease, negating the need for invasive surgery.[62,63]

Small cases series have shown that APC is safe and effective in treating obstructive airway lesions, both malignant and benign.[64–66] It also has been shown to provide benefit in conjunction with chemotherapy in treatment of tuberculosis with evidence of airway lesions.[67] In 1 case series of 364 patients who underwent bronchoscopy for treatment of airway tumors, APC was shown effective in hemostasis control, stent recanalization, and tumor debulking.[64]

Electrocautery

This is a contact modality that uses an electrical probe to direct a monopolar current in to tissue to cause vaporization and coagulation. The probe tip can come in different forms, such as a snare, to loop a polypoid lesion root, or a knife, to cut through fibrotic webs in a stricture.[61] The depth penetration is more superficial compared with a laser, with the risks similar except that no eye protection is required for operation.

Electrocautery has been shown a safe and effective therapy in treating CAO.[61,65,68,69] In a case series of 94 patients who underwent bronchoscopy with electrocautery for malignant or benign disease, endoscopic improvement was seen in 94% of cases along with 78% radiological improvement in luminal patency on CT and, similarly, lung aeration on both CT (63%) and radiograph (43%).[68] A study by Boxem and colleagues[70] showed electrocautery demonstrated comparable efficacy to Nd:YAG laser therapy in the palliative treatment of symptomatic airway obstruction and was significantly more cost effective.

Cryotherapy and Cryoextraction

Conventional cryotherapy involves repeated free-thaw cycles and can be used to treat airway stenosis, granulation tissue recurrence, and early-grade airway lesions.[71] Freezing cells to subzero temperatures using liquid nitrogen induces cell death by damaging blood vessels, causing ischemia. Formation of ice crystals creates an osmotic gradient, driving water out of cells, resulting in cell rupture.

In acute CAO due to endoluminal disease, debulking of exophytic lesions can be performed using cryoextraction (**Fig. 8**A, B). This allows for larger pieces of tissue to be removed, enabling rapid more efficient debulking.[72] The cryoprobe is positioned on to a target area of tumor before freezing. While the probe tip is adhered to tumor, both it and scope are retracted, shearing off larger chunks of tissue. It is effective, with a review of 16 case series demonstrating an overall success rate for significant recanalization of approximately 80%.[73]

Another potential role for cryotherapy is the removal of endobronchial clots causing ventilatory failure secondary to airway obstruction in patients presenting with massive hemoptysis (**Fig. 8**C, D). Often, such patients are critically unwell in an intensive care unit, with mechanical ventilation struggling to compensate. Cryotherapy can be used to remove clots and restore airflow to subsegmental airways, leading to a rapid improvement in clinical state.[74]

BRONCHOSCOPIC RADIOFREQUENCY AND MICROWAVE ABLATION

Experience in percutaneous ablation of lung lesions is well documented in the literature. The RAPTURE trial demonstrated the effectiveness in using radiofrequency ablation (RFA) to treat nonoperable pulmonary or oligometastatic lesions.[75] Microwave ablation (MWA) offers better physical properties with more consistent ablation fields, reduced heat sink effect, and less distortion due to tissue impedance. In one meta-analysis of 53 studies and more than 3000

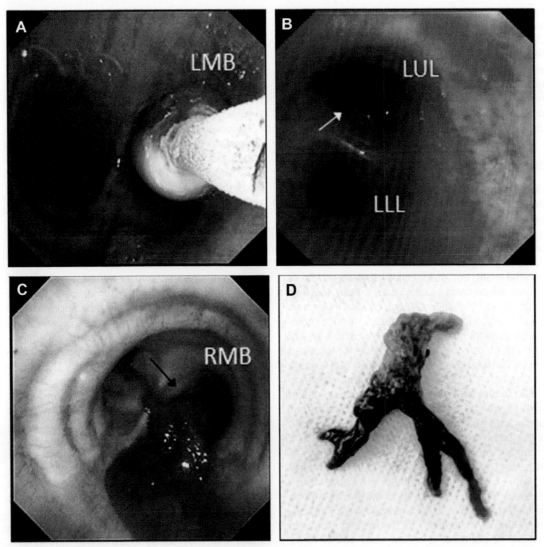

Fig. 8. Bronchoscopic cryoextraction. (*A*) Left main bronchus (LMB) obstruction due to a lesion within the airway; cryoprobe seen freezing on to surface of lesion to begin debulking. (*B*) Successful cryoextraction of the airway lesion to its origin in the left upper lobe (LUL). (*C*) Visible partially organized clot originating from right main bronchus (RMB) and flowing over main carina in to left lung in an intensive care unit patient with massive hemoptysis. (*D*) Sample of clot extracted from subsegmental airway using cryoprobe, which demonstrates an airway cast appearance.

patients, percutaneous application of both modalities in the treatment of pulmonary lesions demonstrated similar efficacy rates, 86% versus 81.1%.[76] The drawbacks of percutaneous approaches, however, remain, in particular, the risk of pneumothorax, which, although quoted at approximately 15% to 20% in some studies, has been observed as high as 50% in others. This has led in some part to a growing interest regarding potential bronchoscopic delivery of thermal ablation to target and treat peripheral lung lesions.

A seminal study on the use of bronchoscopic RFA was carried out on lungs from anesthetized sheep (N = 6) to assess safety and efficacy, followed-up by a similar porcine-based study assessing MWA in the same context.[77,78] The first human pilot evaluated CBCT bronchoscopy and RFA performed in 10 individuals with T1N0M0 lung cancer who subsequently had surgical resection, which demonstrated promising results with no adverse events noted.[79] A similar 20-patient study was carried out by a Chinese research group assessing use of RFA delivered via bronchoscope to treat primary lung tumors, of 24-mm median size. In this group, patients included had T1-2aN0M0 NSCLC, with local tumor control recorded as 82.6% on CT follow-up and 61% 5-year survival.[80] Given the potential promise, this represents an interesting new prospect in the realm of IP. **Table 2** outlines the current trials in progress and the imaging modalities used by the corresponding groups.

ENDOBRONCHIAL BRACHYTHERAPY

Delivery of focused intraluminal high-dose radio-therapy to a tumor bed along an airway wall can be effective in treating, arresting, or slowing disease progression and thereby preventing pending obstruction and collapse (**Fig. 9**).[81–83] This can apply to malignant disease, such as cancer, and nonmalignant but progressive disease, such as airway amyloidosis. Gamma rays from focused radiotherapy (typically iridium) cause DNA chain breaks, triggering cell apoptosis and reduce prolif-eration. The therapeutic effect takes up to 4 weeks to 6 weeks, making it more suitable for localized slowly progressive disease rather than acute obstruction.[71,84] Mediastinitis, esophagitis, and fistula formation are key specific complications of note as well as massive hemoptysis, which may occur after treatment of upper lobe airway lesions with close proximity to pulmonary vessels.

Studies have shown brachytherapy is effective in helping treat clinical symptoms in progressive palliative disease.[81,82,84] In 1 study, 81 patients un-derwent high-dose endobronchial brachytherapy for malignant disease, of which 76 were lung pri-mary and 5 metastatic.[81] Clinical symptoms of cough, hemoptysis, dyspnea, and stridor were seen to improve, with 84.53% of patients experi-encing a complete clinical response and only 1 out of 24 continuing to experience hemoptysis post-treatment. A retrospective review of 88 pa-tients over a 13-year period in Massachusetts saw similar responses and noted survival benefits were best seen in metastatic (nonthoracic origin) lesions, followed by NSCLC.

Although some studies suggest it may be used effectively in combination with external beam radiotherapy or chemotherapy, a Cochrane review in 2012 suggested against this, citing insufficient evidence to suggest brachytherapy combined with external beam radiotherapy or chemotherapy or Nd:YAG laser ablation was more effective.[85]

PHOTODYNAMIC THERAPY

The use of a photosensitizer administered system-atically and retained within tumor cells to allow application of targeted light therapy approximately 2 days later to induce tumor necrosis is well recog-nized. The first reported use of photodynamic ther-apy (PDT) to treat endobronchial lung cancer was in 1980 in a patient who declined surgery and under-went successful ODT with compete remission for the next 4 years. Following this, several reports have outlined its use in treating early and advanced endobronchial disease.[86–88]

PDT can be carried out under topical anesthetic, but general anesthesia often is more preferable. Recognized side effects include skin photosensi-tivity, hemoptysis, cough, and transient dyspnea postprocedure. Repeat bronchoscopy 2 days to 3 days after illumination is advised to assess for possible airway swelling and débride postnecrosis tissue that may cause distal airway obstruction.

Table 2
Current radiofrequency and microwave in progress registered on clinicaltrials.gov

Ablative Modality	Postablation Resection?	Number of Participants	Navigational Method	Region	Clinical Trials Identifier	Sponsor
RFA	No	50	ENB	China	NCT03009630	Shanghai Chest Hospital
RFA	Yes	10	BTPNA	China	NCT03272971	Bronchus Medical; Uptake Medical
RFA/MWA	No	60[a]	ENB	China	NCT02972177	Shanghai Chest Hospital
MWA	No	30	CBCT	USA	NCT03713099	Ethicon
MWA	No	30	CBCT	UK	NCT03569111	Medtronic-MITG
MWA	No	60	ENB	China	NCT04005157	Shanghai Chest Hospital

Abbreviations: BTPNA, bronchoscopic transparenchymal nodule access; ENB, electromagnetic navigational bronchoscopy.
[a] 30 patients in per each modality.

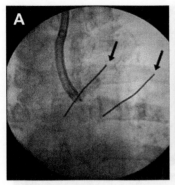 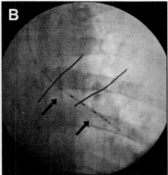

Fig. 9. Intraluminal brachytherapy. (*A*) Bronchoscopic marking of proximal and distal margins of intended airway for treatment; zones then marked superficially (*arrows*) on the patient's chest with skin markers. (*B*) Brachytherapy catheter (*arrows*) inserted using the bronchoscope and positioned carefully in the intended airway segment.

This is more common in exophytic bulky disease rather than mucosal early grade lesions.

In a review of 24 reported case series of PDT to treat either advanced exophytic disease or early-grade lesions, 12 studies outlined use of PDT in symptomatic advanced endoluminal lesions, causing greater than 50% obstruction.[89] Treatment was associated with almost complete symptom relief and correlated with improved spirometry. Factors influencing response related to stage of disease at time of treatment and performance status (>2 associated with a poorer outcome).[90,91] In patients with early-stage bronchial carcinoma, complete response was reported in more than 70% cases. Cure rates were higher in lesions less than 1 cm in diameter, with some newer photosensitizing agents demonstrating better antitumor properties and outcomes for lesions above 1 cm. Addition of adjuvant therapies, such as external beam radiotherapy, was associated with an improved response rate.

PDT also has been shown effective in treating nonbronchogenic endobronchial metastases, with acute relief of hemoptysis and dyspnea seen in 85% of patients in 1 case series.[92] The 30-day mortality, however, was 22% but a majority of cases were renal cell carcinomas, which are notoriously vascular and hazardous to treat endobronchially.

BRONCHOPLASTY AND INTRALESIONAL STEROID INJECTION

Airway strictures can cause significant compromise in patients with high symptom burden. They may develop in the context of active disease, such as vasculitis; after previous airway insults, such as tuberculosis; or as a late complication of previous therapies, for example, PDT and surgery. Management of such strictures can be challenging and is guided best by symptoms, spirometry, and evidence of downstream complications, such as

recurrent infections, high sputum loads, or lobar collapse.

Studies have shown that bronchoscopic balloon dilatation is an effective method to treat airway strictures (**Fig. 10**).[93–95] In cases of high tracheal lesions, advice from a specialist airway otorhinolaryngology team should be sought, and, in some cases, performing bronchoscopy under suspension laryngoscopy may be beneficial.[96] Strictures may be managed through a combination of approaches, such as laser, brachytherapy, and cautery.[97,98] In cases of airway vasculitis, systemic immunosuppression also should be addressed in addition to local treatment of airway disease.

AIRWAY STENTING

The first airway stent was inserted by Harkins[99] in the management of benign tracheal stenosis. Over time, newer stents have been developed and trialed as understanding of bronchial dynamics and airway pathology increases. **Table 3** outlines the variety of stents currently available. More commonly, self-expanding metallic airway stents (SEMAS) are often used and available in a covered design, which is removable if required in the future.

Impending critical airway obstruction, particularly due to extraluminal disease, may require immediate stenting to prevent asphyxia (**Fig. 11**). Symptoms often develop once obstruction is greater than 50%. Where employed, stents should be used as a bridging tool for consolidative therapies (eg, radiotherapy) to treat underlying disease and protect the bronchial tree. If successful, this may allow for stent removal at a later date. Airway stenting can remain unpredictable, however, and careful decision making should be undertaken when weighing up the potential benefits versus risks both short term and long term (**Fig. 12, Table 4**).

Experience in endobronchial stent insertion, although extensively reported in case series,

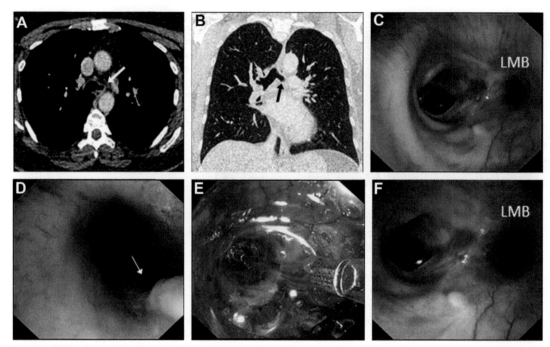

Fig. 10. Balloon bronchoplasty and intra-airway steroid injection. (*A–C*) Left main bronchus (LMB) stricture seen on CT and on bronchoscopy in a patient with vasculitis. (*D*) Injection of methylprednisolone into the airway wall to deliver local anti-inflammatory therapy. (*E*) Noncutting balloon dilatation performed to stretch open the stricture. (*F*) Postintervention endobronchial appearances showing improved luminal diameter of the LMB orifice.

suffers from a lack of objective reported data. Therefore, information is collated from specialist center experiences and accounts of patient cohorts. In 1 large case series, 95% of patients experienced benefit from endobronchial stent insertion for CAO; however, complication rates were notably high, at 42%, with secretion blockage the most common.[100] In 1 retrospective 7-year review of 924 patients who underwent silicone stenting for mixed etiology of CAO, the

Table 3
Types of airway stents and associated features

Type	Features
Silicone	Most commonly used worldwide, able to withstand significant extrinsic forces but disrupts mucus clearance
Montgomery T-tube	Used for subglottic stenosis and requires a tracheal stoma, helpful in laryngeal and high tracheal obstruction, exchangeable/removable
Dumon	Studded wall design visible in radiograph, deployed using rigid bronchoscopy and available in Y-stent shape
Polyflex	Tungsten dotted markers for visibility on radiograph, less prone to granulation but more likely to migrate
Uncovered metallic	Useful in managing extrinsic disease only and not removable; therefore, only for limited expectancy cases Early variants were expandable through bronchoplasty
SEMASs	Made of itinoln alloy; expand postinsertion to final diameter through metal memory/retained elasticity. Prone to metal fatigue
AERO/alveolus	Fully covered nitinol SEMAS, easily removable. Useful in cases of temporary need for stenting to permit other treatment

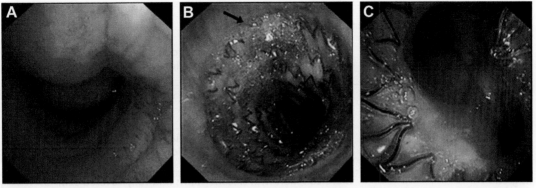

Fig. 11. Tracheal obstruction and airway stenting in an elderly smoker presenting with cough and breathlessness. (*A*) Severe extrinsic compression of the lower trachea seen on bronchoscopy. (*B*) Covered SEMAS inserted, proximal end view showing blue purse string (*arrow*), which can be grasped using forceps to reposition or remove the stent. (*C*) View of distal end of stent with good patency of proximal main bronchi (patient also had mixed obstructive disease in the left main bronchus).

complication rate was 21%, with only 9% due to stent migration.[101] There are numerous reports by groups detailing that stent insertion does help improve quality of life, breathlessness, and lung function but there is variation amongst clinical practice, stent choice, and complication report.

Tracheobronchomalacia and similar entities, such as excessive dynamic airway collapse, are causes of chronic breathlessness that continue to prove difficult to treat, with no consensus on whether stenting is effective. Stenting often is unpredictable and unlikely to prove effective in managing symptoms balanced against side effects and longer-term risks. In 1 study of 58 patients with tracheobronchomalacia who underwent endobronchial stenting, although initial subjective markers of breathlessness and quality of life were noted to improve, this was counterbalanced by no improvement in FEV_1 and significant complications developing as early as 4 weeks postinsertion.[102] Stenting trials with symptom control, improved dynamic CT findings, and spirometry allow for definitive surgical correction in many centers.[103]

Endobronchial stenting may be helpful outside of pending CAO. In cases of aerodigestive fistulas, often seen in locally advanced esophageal cancer, stenting can help seal a fistula and protect against recurrent aspiration and airway insult.[104,105] There have been reports in the literature of stents used to close bronchopleural fistulae and to bridge anastomotic healing in cases of dehiscence.[106,107]

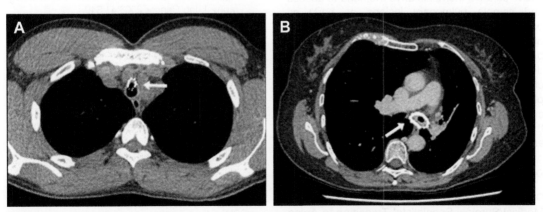

Fig. 12. Airway stenting and complications. (*A*) Patient born with complete tracheal rings, which required surgical fracture as a neonate and bare metal stent insertion–stent fracture over time with partial migration toward great vessels in mediastinum. (*B*) Mucostasis and granulation tissue formation in a patient with a vasculitis-related bronchomalacia of the left main bronchus, which required previous stenting.

Table 4
Potential complications of airway stents

Mucostasis	Most common complication due to impaired mucociliary clearance and tendency for mucus impaction; long-term mucolytic therapy important
Granulation tissue formation	Localized inflammatory response, which may require debulking or steroid injection; most common at proximal and distal stent margins
Bacterial overgrowth	Biofilm formation common, associated with *Staphyloccoccus* and *Pseudomonas*, may require prolonged antibiotics or stent removal/replacement
Migration	More common with silicone stents and fully covered SEMASs Anterior wall suture insertion may be required if high risk
Fracture/fatigue	Rare but due to forces sustained during coughing; some alloys may be less resilient but newer nitinol alloy SEMAS show greater elasticity and durability
Bronchovascular fistula	Rare but possibly more common in specific stent cases with close proximity to hilar and pulmonary anatomy
Airway wall perforation	Less common, previously seen more so with bare metal and first-generation SEMASs

SUMMARY

Recent advancements in the recognition and understanding of both malignant and benign chronic diseases have continued to evolve. The role of IP as a diagnostic and therapeutic tool has become increasingly important given the scope of having a positive impact on diseases and conditions that previously were saturated in their treatment approaches.

Progress in systemic treatment options for malignant disease has resulted in a greater drive toward optimization of symptomatic patients through bronchoscopic intervention in order to enable access to anticancer therapy. Similarly, increased screening and potential identification of early lung cancers combined with newer noninvasive curative therapies drive the need to access and sample pulmonary lesions as early as possible. For this, advanced diagnostic approaches are vital and may in the future offer combination with therapeutic interventions and the delivery of local therapy within the lung parenchyma without the need for other invasive sampling or treatment. IP has been established as critical to optimal diagnosis and management of thoracic disorders and its role is likely to evolve as more therapeutic interventions are evaluated.

DISCLOSURE

Dr S. Shaefi is supported by a Grant for Early Medical/Surgical Specialists' Transition to Aging Research (GEMSSTAR) award (R03AG060179) from the National Institute on Aging and a Mentored Clinical Scientist Research Career Development Award from the National Institute of General Medical Sciences (K08GM134220). This work was undertaken partly at UCLH/UCL, which received a proportion of funding from the Department of Health NIHR Biomedical Research Centre funding stream. Dr N. Navani is supported by a Medical Research Council fellowship (MR/T02481X/1).

REFERENCES

1. Leef JL, Klein JS. The solitary pulmonary nodule. Radiol Clin North Am 2002;40(1):123–43, ix.
2. Midthun DE, Swensen SJ, Jett JR, et al. O-127 Evaluation of nodules detected by screening for lung cancer with low dose spiral computed tomography. Lung Cancer 2003;41:S40.
3. Ost D. The solitary pulmonary nodule. N Engl J Med 2003;348:2535–42.
4. Shulman L, Ost D. Advances in bronchoscopic diagnosis of lung cancer. Curr Opin Pulm Med 2007;13(4):271–7.
5. Vyas KS, Davenport DL, Ferraris VA, et al. Mediastinoscopy: trends and practice patterns in the United States. South Med J 2013;106(10):539–44.
6. Wilson DO, Weissfeld JL, Fuhrman CR, et al. The Pittsburgh Lung Screening Study (PLuSS): outcomes within 3 years of a first computed tomography scan. Am J Respir Crit Care Med 2008;178(9):956–61.
7. Swensen SJ, Jett JR, Hartman TE, et al. CT screening for lung cancer: five-year prospective experience. Radiology 2005;235(1):259–65.

8. Pastorino U, Bellomi M, Landoni C, et al. Early lung-cancer detection with spiral CT and positron emission tomography in heavy smokers: 2-year results. Lancet 2003;362(9384):593–7.

9. Navani N, Brown JM, Nankivell M, et al. Suitability of endobronchial ultrasound-guided transbronchial needle aspiration specimens for subtyping and genotyping of non-small cell lung cancer: a multicenter study of 774 patients. Am J Respir Crit Care Med 2012;185(12):1316–22.

10. Kerr KM, Lamb D, Wathen CG, et al. Pathological assessment of mediastinal lymph nodes in lung cancer: implications for non-invasive mediastinal staging. Thorax 1992;47(5):337–41.

11. Silvestri GA, Gould MK, Margolis ML, et al. Noninvasive staging of non-small cell lung cancer: ACCP evidenced-based clinical practice guidelines (2nd edition). Chest 2007;132(3 Suppl):178S–201S.

12. Silvestri GA, Gonzalez AV, Jantz MA, et al. Methods for staging non-small cell lung cancer: diagnosis and management of lung cancer, 3rd ed: American College of Chest Physicians evidence-based clinical practice guidelines. Chest 2013;143(5 Suppl): e211S–50S.

13. McLoud TC, Bourgouin PM, Greenberg RW, et al. Bronchogenic carcinoma: analysis of staging in the mediastinum with CT by correlative lymph node mapping and sampling. Radiology 1992; 182(2):319–23.

14. Annema JT, van Meerbeeck JP, Rintoul RC, et al. Mediastinoscopy vs endosonography for mediastinal nodal staging of lung cancer: a randomized trial. JAMA 2010;304(20):2245–52.

15. Ernst A, Anantham D, Eberhardt R, et al. Diagnosis of mediastinal adenopathy-real-time endobronchial ultrasound guided needle aspiration versus mediastinoscopy. J Thorac Oncol 2008;3(6):577–82.

16. Navani N, Nankivell M, Lawrence DR, et al. Lung cancer diagnosis and staging with endobronchial ultrasound-guided transbronchial needle aspiration compared with conventional approaches: an open-label, pragmatic, randomised controlled trial. Lancet Respir Med 2015;3(4):282–9.

17. Mondoni M, Sotgiu G, Bonifazi M, et al. Transbronchial needle aspiration in peripheral pulmonary lesions: a systematic review and meta-analysis. Eur Respir J 2016;48(1):196–204.

18. Casal RF, Sarkiss M, Jones AK, et al. Cone beam computed tomography-guided thin/ultrathin bronchoscopy for diagnosis of peripheral lung nodules: a prospective pilot study. J Thorac Dis 2018; 10(12):6950–9.

19. Pritchett MA, Schampaert S, de Groot JAH, et al. Cone-beam CT with augmented fluoroscopy combined with electromagnetic navigation bronchoscopy for biopsy of pulmonary nodules. J Bronchol Interv Pulmonol 2018;25(4):274–82.

20. Hürter T, Hanrath P. Endobronchial sonography: feasibility and preliminary results. Thorax 1992; 47(7):565–7.

21. Herth FJF, Ernst A, Becker HD. Endobronchial ultrasound-guided transbronchial lung biopsy in solitary pulmonary nodules and peripheral lesions. Eur Respir J 2002;20(4):972–4.

22. Jacomelli M, Demarzo SE, Cardoso PFG, et al. Radial-probe EBUS for the diagnosis of peripheral pulmonary lesions. J Bras Pneumol 2016;42(4): 248–53.

23. Steinfort DP, Khor YH, Manser RL, et al. Radial probe endobronchial ultrasound for the diagnosis of peripheral lung cancer: systematic review and meta-analysis. Eur Respir J 2011;37(4):902–10.

24. Ali MS, Trick W, Mba BI, et al. Radial endobronchial ultrasound for the diagnosis of peripheral pulmonary lesions: A systematic review and meta-analysis. Respirol Carlton Vic 2017;22(3): 443–53.

25. Khandhar SJ, Bowling MR, Flandes J, et al. Electromagnetic navigation bronchoscopy to access lung lesions in 1,000 subjects: first results of the prospective, multicenter NAVIGATE study. BMC Pulm Med 2017;17(1):59.

26. Folch EE, Pritchett MA, Nead MA, et al. Electromagnetic navigation bronchoscopy for peripheral pulmonary lesions: one-year results of the prospective, multicenter NAVIGATE study. J Thorac Oncol 2019;14(3):445–58.

27. Bowling MR, Folch EE, Khandhar SJ, et al. Fiducial marker placement with electromagnetic navigation bronchoscopy: a subgroup analysis of the prospective, multicenter NAVIGATE study. Ther Adv Respir Dis 2019;13. 1753466619841234.

28. Herth FJF, Eberhardt R, Sterman D, et al. Bronchoscopic transparenchymal nodule access (BTPNA): first in human trial of a novel procedure for sampling solitary pulmonary nodules. Thorax 2015; 70(4):326–32.

29. Harzheim D, Sterman D, Shah PL, et al. Bronchoscopic transparenchymal nodule access: feasibility and safety in an endoscopic unit. Respir Int Rev Thorac Dis 2016;91(4):302–6.

30. Mondoni M, Sotgiu G. Bronchoscopic management of peripheral pulmonary lesions: robotic approach paves the way to the future. BMC Pulm Med 2019;19(1):166.

31. Chen AC, Gillespie CT. Robotic endoscopic airway challenge: REACH assessment. Ann Thorac Surg 2018;106(1):293–7.

32. Rojas-Solano JR, Ugalde-Gamboa L, Machuzak M. Robotic bronchoscopy for diagnosis of suspected lung cancer: a feasibility study. J Bronchol Interv Pulmonol 2018;25(3):168–75.

33. Lee P, van den Berg RM, Lam S, et al. Color fluorescence ratio for detection of bronchial dysplasia

and carcinoma in situ. Clin Cancer Res 2009;
15(14):4700–5.

34. Zhang J, Wu J, Yang Y, et al. White light, autofluorescence and narrow-band imaging bronchoscopy
for diagnosing airway pre-cancerous and early
cancer lesions: a systematic review and meta-analysis. J Thorac Dis 2016;8(11):3205–16.

35. Lam B, Lam SY, Wong MP, et al. Sputum cytology
examination followed by autofluorescence bronchoscopy: a practical way of identifying early stage
lung cancer in central airway. Lung Cancer 2009;
64(3):289–94.

36. Zaric B, Stojsic V, Sarcev T, et al. Advanced bronchoscopic techniques in diagnosis and staging of
lung cancer. J Thorac Dis 2013;5(Suppl 4):
S359–70.

37. Sun J, Garfield DH, Lam B, et al. The value of autofluorescence bronchoscopy combined with white
light bronchoscopy compared with white light
alone in the diagnosis of intraepithelial neoplasia
and invasive lung cancer: a meta-analysis.
J Thorac Oncol 2011;6(8):1336–44.

38. Epelbaum O, Aronow WS. Autofluorescence bronchoscopy for lung cancer screening: a time to
reflect. Ann Transl Med 2016;4(16):311.

39. Iftikhar IH, Musani AI. Narrow-band imaging bronchoscopy in the detection of premalignant airway
lesions: a meta-analysis of diagnostic test accuracy. Ther Adv Respir Dis 2015;9(5):207–16.

40. Shibuya K, Nakajima T, Fujiwara T, et al. Narrow
band imaging with high-resolution bronchovideo-
scopy: a new approach for visualizing angiogenesis in squamous cell carcinoma of the lung.
Lung Cancer Amst Neth 2010;69(2):194–202.

41. Herth FJF, Eberhardt R, Anantham D, et al. Narrow-
band imaging bronchoscopy increases the specificity of bronchoscopic early lung cancer detection.
J Thorac Oncol 2009;4(9):1060–5.

42. Advani M, Purohit G, Vyas S, et al. Comparison of
diagnostic potential of narrow band imaging bronchoscopy over white light bronchoscopy in lung
cancer. J Bronchol Interv Pulmonol 2018;25(2):
132–6.

43. Zhu J, Li W, Zhou J, et al. The diagnostic value of
narrow-band imaging for early and invasive lung
cancer: a meta-analysis. Clinics (Sao Paulo)
2017;72(7):438–48.

44. Babiak A, Hetzel J, Krishna G, et al. Transbronchial
cryobiopsy: a new tool for lung biopsies. Respir Int
Rev Thorac Dis 2009;78(2):203–8.

45. Griff S, Ammenwerth W, Schönfeld N, et al. Mor-
phometrical analysis of transbronchial cryobiopsies. Diagn Pathol 2011;6:53.

46. Han Q, Luo Q, Xie J-X, et al. Diagnostic yield and
postoperative mortality associated with surgical
lung biopsy for evaluation of interstitial lung diseases: A systematic review and meta-analysis.

J Thorac Cardiovasc Surg 2015;149(5):1394–401.
e1.

47. Johannson KA, Marcoux VS, Ronksley PE, et al.
Diagnostic yield and complications of transbron-
chial lung cryobiopsy for interstitial lung disease.
A systematic review and metaanalysis. Ann Am
Thorac Soc 2016;13(10):1828–38.

48. Ravaglia C, Bonifazi M, Wells AU, et al. Safety and
diagnostic yield of transbronchial lung cryobiopsy
in diffuse parenchymal lung diseases: a comparative study versus video-assisted thoracoscopic
lung biopsy and a systematic review of the literature. Respir Int Rev Thorac Dis 2016;91(3):215–27.

49. Tomassetti S, Wells AU, Costabel U, et al. Bronchoscopic lung cryobiopsy increases diagnostic confidence in the multidisciplinary diagnosis of
idiopathic pulmonary fibrosis. Am J Respir Crit
Care Med 2016;193(7):745–52.

50. Romagnoli M, Colby TV, Berthet J-P, et al. Poor
concordance between sequential transbronchial
lung cryobiopsy and surgical lung biopsy in the
diagnosis of diffuse interstitial lung diseases. Am
J Respir Crit Care Med 2019;199(10):1249–56.

51. Troy LK, Grainge C, Corte TJ, et al. Diagnostic accuracy of transbronchial lung cryobiopsy for interstitial
lung disease diagnosis (COLDICE): a prospective,
comparative study. Lancet Respir Med 2019.
https://doi.org/10.1016/S2213-2600(19)30342-X.

52. Cavaliere S, Venuta F, Foccoli P, et al. Endoscopic
treatment of malignant airway obstructions in 2,008
patients. Chest 1996;110(6):1536–42.

53. Khemasuwan D, Mehta AC, Wang K-P. Past, present, and future of endobronchial laser photoresection. J Thorac Dis 2015;7(Suppl 4):S380–8.

54. Desai SJ, Mehta AC, VanderBrug Medendorp S,
et al. Survival experience following Nd:YAG laser
photoresection for primary bronchogenic carcinoma. Chest 1988;94(5):939–44.

55. Jang TW, Blackman G, George JJ. Survival benefits of lung cancer patients undergoing laser and
brachytherapy. J Korean Med Sci 2002;17(3):
341–7.

56. Dalar L, Ozdemir C, Abul Y, et al. Endobronchial
treatment of carcinoid tumors of the lung. Thorac
Cardiovasc Surg 2016;64(2):166–71.

57. Neyman K, Sundset A, Naalsund A, et al. Endoscopic treatment of bronchial carcinoids in comparison to surgical resection: a retrospective
study. J Bronchol Interv Pulmonol 2012;19(1):
29–34.

58. Fuks L, Fruchter O, Amital A, et al. Long-term
follow-up of flexible bronchoscopic treatment for
bronchial carcinoids with curative intent. Diagn
Ther Endosc 2009;2009:782961.

59. Goldman L, editor. The biomedical laser. New York:
Springer; 1981. https://doi.org/10.1007/978-1-
4612-5922-0.

60. Grund KE, Storek D, Farin G. Endoscopic argon plasma coagulation (APC) first clinical experiences in flexible endoscopy. Endosc Surg Allied Technol 1994;2(1):42–6.

61. Bolliger CT, Sutedja TG, Strausz J, et al. Therapeutic bronchoscopy with immediate effect: laser, electrocautery, argon plasma coagulation and stents. Eur Respir J 2006;27(6):1258–71.

62. Reddy C, Majid A, Michaud G, et al. Gas embolism following bronchoscopic argon plasma coagulation: a case series. Chest 2008;134(5):1066–9.

63. Shaw Y, Yoneda KY, Chan AL. Cerebral gas embolism from bronchoscopic argon plasma coagulation: a case report. Respir Int Rev Thorac Dis 2012;83(3):267–70.

64. Reichle G, Freitag L, Kullmann HJ, et al. [Argon plasma coagulation in bronchology: a new method–alternative or complementary?]. Pneumol Stuttg Ger 2000;54(11):508–16.

65. Farhat AA, Ragab M, Abd-Elzaher AH, et al. Bronchoscopic electrocauterization versus argon plasma coagulation as a palliative management for patients with bronchogenic carcinoma. Egypt J Chest Dis Tuberc 2015;64(1):243–8.

66. Morice RC, Ece T, Ece F, et al. Endobronchial argon plasma coagulation for treatment of hemoptysis and neoplastic airway obstruction. Chest 2001;119(3):781–7.

67. Jin F, Mu D, Xie Y, et al. Application of bronchoscopic argon plasma coagulation in the treatment of tumorous endobronchial tuberculosis: historical controlled trial. J Thorac Cardiovasc Surg 2013;145(6):1650–3.

68. Wahidi MM, Unroe MA, Adlakha N, et al. The use of electrocautery as the primary ablation modality for malignant and benign airway obstruction. J Thorac Oncol 2011;6(9):1516–20.

69. van Boxem TJ, Westerga J, Venmans BJ, et al. Tissue effects of bronchoscopic electrocautery: bronchoscopic appearance and histologic changes of bronchial wall after electrocautery. Chest 2000;117(3):887–91.

70. Boxem TV, Muller M, Venmans B, et al. Nd-YAG laser vs bronchoscopic electrocautery for palliation of symptomatic airway obstruction: a cost-effectiveness study. Chest 1999;116(4):1108–12.

71. Vergnon J-M, Huber RM, Moghissi K. Place of cryotherapy, brachytherapy and photodynamic therapy in therapeutic bronchoscopy of lung cancers. Eur Respir J 2006;28(1):200–18.

72. Hetzel M, Hetzel J, Schumann C, et al. Cryorecanalization: a new approach for the immediate management of acute airway obstruction. J Thorac Cardiovasc Surg 2004;127(5):1427–31.

73. Lee S-H, Choi W-J, Sung S-W, et al. Endoscopic cryotherapy of lung and bronchial tumors: a systematic review. Korean J Intern Med 2011;26(2):137–44.

74. Lee H, Leem CS, Lee JH, et al. Successful removal of endobronchial blood clots using bronchoscopic cryotherapy at bedside in the intensive care unit. Tuberc Respir Dis (Seoul) 2014;77(4):193–6.

75. Lencioni R, Crocetti L, Cioni R, et al. Response to radiofrequency ablation of pulmonary tumours: a prospective, intention-to-treat, multicentre clinical trial (the RAPTURE study). Lancet Oncol 2008;9(7):621–8.

76. Yuan Z, Wang Y, Zhang J, et al. A meta-analysis of clinical outcomes after radiofrequency ablation and microwave ablation for lung cancer and pulmonary metastases. J Am Coll Radiol 2019;16(3):302–14.

77. Tsushima K, Koizumi T, Tanabe T, et al. Bronchoscopy-guided radiofrequency ablation as a potential novel therapeutic tool. Eur Respir J 2007;29(6):1193–200.

78. Ferguson J, Egressy K, Schefelker R, et al. Bronchoscopically-guided microwave ablation in the lung. Chest 2013;144(4):87A.

79. Tanabe T, Koizumi T, Tsushima K, et al. Comparative study of three different catheters for CT imaging-bronchoscopy-guided radiofrequency ablation as a potential and novel interventional therapy for lung cancer. Chest 2010;137(4):890–7.

80. Koizumi T, Tsushima K, Tanabe T, et al. Bronchoscopy-guided cooled radiofrequency ablation as a novel intervention therapy for peripheral lung cancer. Respir Int Rev Thorac Dis 2015;90(1):47–55.

81. Escobar-Sacristán JA, Granda-Orive JI, Gutiérrez Jiménez T, et al. Endobronchial brachytherapy in the treatment of malignant lung tumours. Eur Respir J 2004;24(3):348–52.

82. Skowronek J. Brachytherapy in the treatment of lung cancer - a valuable solution. J Contemp Brachytherapy 2015;7(4):297–311.

83. Nori D, Allison R, Kaplan B, et al. High dose-rate intraluminal irradiation in bronchogenic carcinoma. Technique and results. Chest 1993;104(4):1006–11.

84. Hardavella G, George J. Interventional bronchoscopy in the management of thoracic malignancy. Breathe (Sheff) 2015;11(3):202–12.

85. Reveiz L, Rueda J-R, Cardona AF. Palliative endobronchial brachytherapy for non-small cell lung cancer. Cochrane Database Syst Rev 2012;(12):CD004284.

86. Moghissi K, Bond MG, Sambrook RJ, et al. Treatment of endotracheal or endobronchial obstruction by non-small cell lung cancer: lack of patients in an MRC randomized trial leaves key questions unanswered. Medical Research Council Lung Cancer Working Party. Clin Oncol (R Coll Radiol) 1999;11(3):179–83.

87. Usuda J, Kato H, Okunaka T, et al. Photodynamic therapy (PDT) for lung cancers. J Thorac Oncol 2006;1(5):489–93.

88. Usuda J, Ichinose S, Ishizumi T, et al. Management of multiple primary lung cancer in patients with centrally located early cancer lesions. J Thorac Oncol 2010;5(1):62–8.

89. Moghissi K, Dixon K. Is bronchoscopic photodynamic therapy a therapeutic option in lung cancer? Eur Respir J 2003;22(3):535–41.

90. McCaughan JS, Williams TE. Photodynamic therapy for endobronchial malignant disease: A prospective fourteen-year study. J Thorac Cardiovasc Surg 1997;114(6):940–7.

91. Moghissi K, Dixon K, Stringer M, et al. The place of bronchoscopic photodynamic therapy in advanced unresectable lung cancer: experience of 100 cases1. Eur J Cardiothorac Surg 1999; 15(1):1–6.

92. Litle VR, Luketich JD, Christie NA, et al. Photodynamic therapy as palliation for esophageal cancer: experience in 215 patients. Ann Thorac Surg 2003; 76(5):1687–92 [discussion: 1692–3].

93. Jabbardarjani HR, Kiani A, Sheikhi N, et al. Balloon bronchoplasty: case series. Tanaffos 2012;11(2): 42–8.

94. Li S. [Interventional management of benign airway stenosis]. Zhonghua Jie He He Hu Xi Za Zhi 2011; 34(5):329–32.

95. Shitrit D, Kuchuk M, Zismanov V, et al. Bronchoscopic balloon dilatation of tracheobronchial stenosis: long-term follow-up. Eur J Cardiothorac Surg 2010;38(2):198–202.

96. Nouraei SAR, Mills H, Butler CR, et al. Outcome of treating airway compromise due to bronchial stenosis with intralesional corticosteroids and cutting-balloon bronchoplasty. Otolaryngol Head Neck Surg 2011;145(4):623–7.

97. Rahman NA, Fruchter O, Shitrit D, et al. Flexible bronchoscopic management of benign tracheal stenosis: long term follow-up of 115 patients. J Cardiothorac Surg 2010;5:2.

98. Garg M, Gogia P, Manoria P, et al. Bronchoscopic management of benign bronchial stenosis by electrocautery and balloon dilatation. Indian J Chest Dis Allied Sci 2012;54(1):41–3.

99. Harkins WB. An endotracheal metallic prosthesis in the treatment of stenosis of the upper trachea. Ann Otol Rhinol Laryngol 1952;61(3):663–76.

100. Wood DE. Airway stenting. Chest Surg Clin N Am 2001;11(4):841–60.

101. Dumon J-F, Cavaliere S, Diaz-Jimenez JP, et al. Seven-year experience with the dumon prosthesis. J Bronchol 1996;3(1):6–10.

102. Ernst A, Majid A, Feller-Kopman D, et al. Airway stabilization with silicone stents for treating adult tracheobronchomalacia: a prospective observational study. Chest 2007;132(2):609–16.

103. Parikh M, Wilson J, Majid A, et al. Airway stenting in excessive central airway collapse. J Vis Surg 2017; 3:172.

104. Herth FJF, Peter S, Baty F, et al. Combined airway and oesophageal stenting in malignant airway-oesophageal fistulas: a prospective study. Eur Respir J 2010;36(6):1370–4.

105. Zhou C, Hu Y, Xiao Y, et al. Current treatment of tracheoesophageal fistula. Ther Adv Respir Dis 2017; 11(4):173–80.

106. de Lima A, Holden V, Gesthalter Y, et al. Treatment of persistent bronchopleural fistula with a manually modified endobronchial stent: a case-report and brief literature review. J Thorac Dis 2018;10(10): 5960–3.

107. Tufail M, Pannu K, Bhusari S, et al. Management of post-pneumonectomy bronchopleural fistula using a Y dumon tracheobronchial stent and a novel deployment technique - a case report. Am J Respir Crit Care Med 2017;2017:A1632.

Section C: Postoperative management

Pain Management in Thoracic Surgery

Kyle Marshall, MD*, Keleigh McLaughlin, MD

KEYWORDS

- Thoracic epidural • Pain • Thoracic surgery • Paravertebral block • Serratus anterior plane block
- Erector spinae plane block

KEY POINTS

- Recognize the sources of pain after thoracic surgery.
- Appreciate the usefulness of multimodal analgesia after thoracic surgery.
- Describe regional anesthesia options for patients undergoing thoracic surgery.
- Incorporate regional and multimodal analgesia into Enhanced Recovery After Surgery protocols.

INTRODUCTION

Thoracic surgery ranks as one of the most painful surgical procedures. Pain after these procedures can be debilitating and lead to poor outcomes, including respiratory complications such as atelectasis and pneumonia, as well as longer hospital stays, poor quality of life, and chronic persistent postoperative pain syndrome.

The most frequent sources of pain after these procedures include surgical incision, rib damage or resection, surgical drains and chest tubes, and the suturing technique. There are many analgesic options for patients undergoing thoracic surgery, including systemic agents and regional anesthesia. A multimodal analgesic approach is thought to be the most effective way to treat these patients.

THORACOTOMY PAIN

Pathophysiology

Pain is mediated via nociceptive somatic and visceral mechanisms, neuropathic mechanisms, as well as referred pain from the phrenic nerve.

Nociceptive somatic afferents are the main source of pain for patients and arise from the intercostal nerves, activated by damage to the chest wall and pleura. Skin incision, trocar insertion,

muscle splitting, rib retraction, and chest tubes or surgical drains contribute to this pain. The signal is transmitted from the intercostal nerve to the ipsilateral dorsal horn of the spinal cord, then to the contralateral anterolateral system, whereby it ascends to the limbic system and somatosensory cortices.[1–3]

Inflammatory mediators, including prostaglandins, bradykinin, histamine, and potassium, are released from the site of injury and directly activate nociceptive receptors. This activation leads to an increased response by the nociceptive receptors, called primary sensitization. If this repeated activation continues, hyperexcitability of the dorsal horn neuron occurs, resulting in release of glutamate, which activates N-methyl-D-aspartate (NMDA) receptors in the spinal cord. The activation of NMDA receptors causes the spinal cord neurons to become more responsive to its inputs, leading to central sensitization.[2] Not only does NMDA receptor activation increase the cell's response to painful stimuli, it also decreases the neuronal sensitivity to opioid receptor agonists.[4]

Nociceptive visceral afferents arise from the vagal nerve as receive nociceptive impulses from the lung, mediastinum, and mediastinal pleura, while the phrenic nerve receives impulses from the diaphragmatic pleura. The referred pain from

University of Colorado Anschutz Medical Campus, 12401 East 17th Avenue, Mail Stop B113, Aurora, CO 80045, USA
* Corresponding author.
E-mail address: kyle.marshall@ucdenver.edu

Thorac Surg Clin 30 (2020) 339–346
https://doi.org/10.1016/j.thorsurg.2020.03.001
1547-4127/20/Published by Elsevier Inc.

the phrenic nerve is often felt in the shoulder and is not relieved by thoracic epidurals, owing to its origination at cervical roots.[3–5]

Neuropathic pain can result from direct injury to the intercostal nerves, and may lead to hypersensitivity and neuralgia, including dysesthesia, allodynia, hyperalgesia, and hyperpathia.[2]

Surgical Risk Factors

Thoracic surgery is typically performed via the classical thoracotomy, minithoracotomy, video-assisted thoracoscopic surgery (VATS), and most recently robot-assisted thoracoscopic surgery (RATS). The classical thoracotomy is a posterolateral incision that allows for optimal surgical access. However, it is also known to be the most painful, because it involves splitting the latissimus dorsi, serratus anterior, rhomboids, and trapezius muscles. Thoracotomy approach has been found to be a major risk factor for the development of new persistent opioid use in thoracic surgery patients.[5]

Minithoracotomy incisions are intended to spare muscle splitting. The result is a decreased field of vision for the surgeon, increasing the risk for excessive rib retraction, dislocation, and damage to the intercostal nerves. In addition, this technique often spans several dermatomes rather than 1 dermatome, as seen in the classical thoracotomy.[1,2]

VATS has increased in popularity because it offers advantages that include smaller incisions, shorter hospital stays, and less postoperative pain. The insertion of trocars can still damage intercostal nerves.[3,6] RATS has become more prevalent in the last decade, with the advantage of allowing surgeons improved ergonomics and wristed instrument motions as well as 3-dimensional views, compared with VATS.

Several retrospective studies have shown RATS to have a longer operative time compared with VATS and open thoracotomies. This disadvantage may be balanced by research suggesting that conversion from RATS to open procedures were decreased as compared with conversion of VATS to open thoracotomy owing to the lower incidence of complications such as bleeding.[7,8] VATS and RATS have not demonstrated significant differences in postoperative pain scores.[9,10]

Patient Risk Factors

Patient factors thought to independently increase pain intensity after surgery include female sex and younger age, although these factors have not been thoroughly studied in thoracic surgery specifically. Patients taking opioids preoperatively have a tolerance and will not benefit from opioids postoperatively to the same degree as opioid-naïve patients.[3]

PAIN MANAGEMENT

Managing pain after thoracic surgery is best addressed with multimodal pharmacologic agents in conjunction with regional anesthesia.

Systemic

Systemic analgesics include nonsteroidal anti-inflammatory drugs (NSAIDs), NMDA receptor antagonists, acetaminophen, gabapentinoids and opioids.

Nonsteroidal anti-inflammatory drugs
NSAIDs are effective adjuncts for analgesia following thoracic surgery. NSAIDs inhibit the cyclo-oxygenase enzyme, therefore decreasing prostaglandin, prostacyclin, and thromboxane synthesis.[11,12] Commonly used NSAIDs include oral meloxicam, ibuprofen, and naproxen, as well as intravenous ketorolac. NSAIDs have been shown to have an additive analgesic effect when combined with other agents. They also effectively treat referred shoulder pain that is, not blocked by a thoracic epidural.[3]

The inhibition of cyclo-oxygenase enzymes has several adverse effects. In the gastrointestinal system, decreased prostaglandin results in increased gastric acid secretion, decreased bicarbonate secretion, and decreased mucin secretion that contribute to damage of the mucosal lining and resulting in the increased the risk of peptic ulcers and bleeding. Prostaglandin inhibition causes renal vasoconstriction. In those with preexisting renal, hepatic, or cardiac disease or volume depletion, this inhibition can lead to acute renal failure.[13] NSAIDs may cause temporary platelet dysfunction and therefore increase the risk of systemic bleeding; however, this factor has not been found to be significant in thoracic surgery.[3] When administering NSAIDs, it is important to take into account the patient's comorbidities and medications to minimize adverse effects. The benefits of improved analgesia and opioid minimization often outweigh the risks of these medications.

N-methyl-D-aspartate antagonist
Ketamine is an NMDA receptor antagonist that provides profound analgesia and decreased inflammatory cytokine release in subanesthetic doses. There are significant side effects in higher doses, including dissociation, hallucination, sympathetic excitation, and cardiac depression. In

contrast with opioids, ketamine does not cause respiratory depression.

Ketamine has been demonstrated to be a valuable adjunct in an opioid-sparing perioperative analgesic plan, achieving lower post-thoracotomy pain scores without a significant increase in adverse events when compared with opioid-only patient-controlled analgesia.[14–17] Additionally, there is evidence of improved oxygenation and ventilation when patient-controlled analgesia with morphine and ketamine was compared with patient-controlled analgesia with morphine alone.[16] Thus far, perioperative ketamine administration has not demonstrated a reduction in the development of chronic post-thoracotomy pain syndrome (PTPS).[17]

Acetaminophen

The exact mechanism of action of acetaminophen on pain receptors is unknown; however, it does inhibit prostaglandin synthesis centrally, where it exerts analgesic and antipyretic effects. Acetaminophen may exert peripheral anti-inflammatory actions, although compared with NSAIDS, the effect is minimal.[18] A recent meta-analysis demonstrated that administration of acetaminophen decreases opioid consumption by up to 20% in thoracic surgery.[19] Acetaminophen is very safe at clinical doses and has few contraindications. It is primarily metabolized by the liver, and caution should be taken when administering to patients with significant liver disease, because one of the metabolites, N-acetyl-p-benzoquinone imine, can lead to liver toxicity.[20]

Gabapentinoids

Commonly used gabapentinoids for neuropathic analgesia include pregabalin and gabapentin. These agents act as GABA analogues, blocking $\alpha2\delta$ subunit-c voltage-dependent calcium channels and providing neuropathic analgesia. A recent meta-analysis evaluated pregabalin's effects on postoperative pain scores, neuropathic pain, and morphine consumption.[21] Their findings indicate that pregabalin significantly reduced visual analog scale (VAS) pain scores at 1 and 3 days and 1 and 3 months, while decreasing postoperative neuropathic pain and morphine consumption to a small extent. Studies determining chronic postoperative pain after thoracotomy found that pregabalin was effective in treating chronic neuropathic pain.

Gabapentinoids have a safe pharmacologic profile; however, their side effects include drowsiness, fatigue, and dizziness. One study found that pregabalin reduced postoperative nausea and vomiting, most likely secondary to decreased opioid consumption. Gabapentinoids are an effective adjunct for thoracic surgery, especially for decreasing postoperative neuropathic pain.

Opioids

Opioids are most commonly administered via intravenous, intrathecal, epidural, oral, or transdermal routes. Opioid-based intravenous patient-controlled analgesia has been widely used for its analgesic efficacy in treating thoracic pain. However, the use of intravenous opioids has shifted from being the primary analgesic to a rescue agent in thoracic surgery. This change is due to the narrow therapeutic window, addiction profile, and detrimental side effects, including respiratory depression, sputum retention, somnolence, constipation, nausea, and vomiting.[1]

The opioid epidemic has received more attention in the last several years as the public has become more aware of opioid dependence and the number of deaths related to opioid overdose. It is estimated that, in 2017, there were more than 49,000 deaths in the United States related to opioid overdose.[22] Physicians have taken the initiative in decreasing opioid prescribing by using multimodal analgesia options.

Preemptive administration of analgesics

Administering preoperative analgesia before noxious stimuli is thought to decrease postoperative pain by preventing the development of altered processing of afferent input and the amplification of postoperative pain.[23] This concept applies to both systemic and regional techniques. In a systematic review of thoracic patients, preoperative thoracic epidural analgesia (TEA) was found to decrease acute postoperative pain, although at 6 months there was no difference in the incidence of chronic pain compared with those receiving TEA after surgery.[24] Another systematic review demonstrated no difference in acute and chronic pain scores with the preemptive administration of NSAIDS, intravenous opioids, or NMDA antagonists.[25] Despite the lack of strong evidence regarding preemptive analgesia, the clinicians continue to administer preoperative analgesia.

Regional Anesthesia

Thoracic epidural analgesia

TEA involves placing a small catheter into the epidural space for neuraxial analgesia. The catheter should be placed at or near the dermatomal level of the surgery. Medications injected through the catheter act on the dorsal column, spinothalamic tract, dorsal and ventral rami, spinal nerve roots, and sympathetic chain.

TEA has long been the gold standard of procedural multimodal analgesia for thoracotomy. It has demonstrated consistent superiority over systemic opioids with pulmonary function and analgesia. Patients with TEA have reduced splinting and improved mucociliary clearance. One reason for this is that TEA is capable of covering several bilateral dermatomal levels.

Common side effects of TEA include hypotension, light headedness, and pruritus. There is also the potential for epidural failure if the catheter tip is in the wrong location or, more commonly, patients receiving a 1-sided or patchy pain relief. Also, attention must be paid to the American Society of Regional Anesthesia guidelines regarding TEA placement and anticoagulation so that catastrophic complications such as epidural hematoma can be avoided.[26]

TEA has been shown in a meta-analysis to be similar to continuous paravertebral nerve block (PVB) for pain scores and opioid sparing, but with more minor side effects.[27] However, there are still new studies that state improved pain with TEA when compared with PVB.[28,29] One consistent downside of TEA remains systemic hypotension.

Intercostal nerve block

The intercostal nerve block (ICNB) is often placed by the surgeon under direct visualization of the nerve bundle at the conclusion of the case as an adjunct in multimodal post-thoracotomy analgesia. The block is performed by injecting a local anesthetic near the intercostal nerves, at multiple levels, and with 3 to 5 mL of local anesthetic deposited per block. Unilateral, single-level analgesia is produced by each injection.

ICNB is infrequently performed by anesthesiologists for several reasons. Adequate blockade requires 5 or 6 single shot injections for broad dermatomal coverage. If not done under direct visualization, each subsequent injection presents a risk of pneumothorax, nerve injury, and vascular damage. Systemic absorption of local anesthetic is high at the intercostal location, making analgesia short lived and the risk of local anesthetic systemic toxicity higher than other options. Continuous and single shot ICNB techniques have been shown to be superior to systemic opioids alone.[30,31] However, intercostal nerve catheters have been found to be inferior to TEA.[30]

New promise for long-duration ICNB has come with the advent of liposomal bupivacaine. A few small studies have shown similar, and even better analgesia in some instances than TEA up to 72 hours after ICNB placement.[32,33] Further research continues comparing long-acting bupivacaine with thoracic wall blocks, PVB and TEA.

Paravertebral nerve block

The PVB is an effective block that can cause sympathetic and somatic blockade ipsilaterally via injectate close to the thoracic spinal nerves emerging from the intervertebral foramen. The paravertebral space is a potential space lateral to the vertebral column, posterior to the parietal pleura, and anterior to the costotransverse ligament. Placement can be either percutaneous using ultrasound guidance, or intraoperatively with surgeons placing a single shot or catheter under direct visualization. When performing percutaneous placement, the needle is inserted perpendicular to the skin, approximately 3 cm lateral to the spinous process, and is advanced until contact is made with the transverse process. The needle is then walked off the cephalad edge of the transverse process and slowly advanced until a loss of resistance is encountered, typically 1 cm deeper than the transverse process. A single shot can be performed or a catheter may be placed.[3] Often, PVB requires several injections to obtain sufficient dermatomes, most commonly at the T3, T5, and T7 levels.

As discussed elsewhere in this article, studies have demonstrated excellent analgesia comparable with TEA with fewer side effects such as hypotension.[3,6,27] The paravertebral space remains a noncompressible area and American Society of Regional Anesthesia guidelines regarding anticoagulation should be strictly followed.[26] Experience with PVB influences the success of these blocks and is largely institution and physician dependent.

Intrathecal blockade

Intrathecal administration of opioids is an infrequent but effective method of providing post-thoracotomy analgesia for approximately 24 hours.[2,3] Intrathecal administration is performed in the lumbar region, with opioids spreading cephalad in the cerebrospinal fluid and binding to opioid receptors of the dorsal horn. Depending on the chosen opioid, the onset and duration of analgesia is affected. Hydrophilic opioids such as morphine have a slower onset of action; however, entry into the circulation is delayed, allowing for a longer duration. Side effects of intrathecal opioid administration are much less severe than systemic opioid administration, but does include nausea and vomiting, respiratory depression, pruritus, and urinary retention.[34]

Erector spinae plane block

Erector spinae plane (ESP) block is a recently described plane block that involves depositing local anesthetic deep to the erector spinae muscle (longissimus thoracis), but superficial to the transverse process (**Fig. 1**). The block should be performed at the level of T4 for thoracic surgery. ESP block should be done under ultrasound guidance, to see the cephalocaudad spread of local anesthetic and to verify that the needle has emerged from the erector spinae muscle fascia. Injectate acts on the ventral and dorsal rami of the spinal cord from spread to the paravertebral and epidural spaces, as well as posterior and lateral cutaneous intercostal nerves on chest wall, resulting in analgesia over the hemithorax. The block is capable of covering dermatomes T2 to T10; however, this depends on dermatomal level placement and volume injected. ESP may be performed as a single shot or continuous technique.

ESP block may be considered for preemptive or rescue analgesia, with preemptive analgesia considered for intraoperative opioid sparing. The block has a low risk profile, because it is not close to the pleura, spinal cord, nerves, or major blood vessels. It is safer with anticoagulation than neuraxial techniques (TEA, PVB) and avoids potential catastrophic consequences such as epidural hematoma.[35]

ESP block has shown comparable analgesia and less side effects to PVB.[36] It has demonstrated effective pain control and limited complications in patients on anticoagulation receiving left ventricular assist devices via left thoracotomy.[37] A small case series has also shown ESP block efficacy after VATS procedures, as well as rescue after orthotopic lung transplantation.[38] The block has also shown promise in patients with PTPS, improving pain weeks after surgery

and causing prolonged analgesia for some after single shot block.[39]

Serratus anterior block

The serratus anterior plane (SAP) block is another plane block that requires local anesthetic deposition either deep or superficial to the serratus anterior muscle, at the midaxillary line, anywhere from ribs 2 to 7 (**Fig. 2**). Similar to an ESP block, a SAP block may be single shot or continuous technique and may be placed preemptively or as a rescue block. Postoperative rescue block or catheter placement can be difficult because of the surgical site dressing and unpredictable injectate spread after surgical violation of the muscle plane. SAP block affects the lateral intercostal nerves, with anterior and posterior dermatomal spread around T2 to T9; however, it depends on thoracic-level placement, continuity of tissue plane, and volume injected.[35]

SAP block has a low risk profile, because it is not close to major blood vessels, nerves, or pleura. Long thoracic and thoracodorsal nerves may also be blocked by the injectate. A SAP block is considered safer in anticoagulated patients than neuraxial procedures (TEA, PVB) and is an easily compressible area, in the event of hematoma. Similar to an ESP block, it also avoids devastating neuraxial injuries.

The SAP block has been shown to decrease VAS scores and morphine consumption, in comparison with intravenous opioids with NSAIDs and acetaminophen, up to 24 hours after single-shot placement. This subset also showed a decrease in postoperative nausea and vomiting.[40]

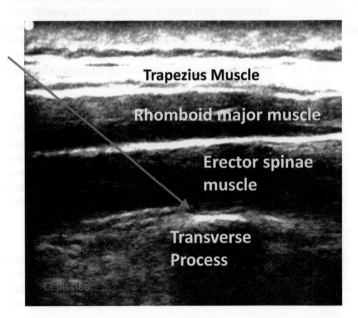

Fig. 1. Ultrasound image depicts the anatomy for ESP block. The *orange line* indicates the trajectory of the block needle.

Trapezius Muscle

Rhomboid major muscle

Erector spinae muscle

Transverse Process

Cephalad

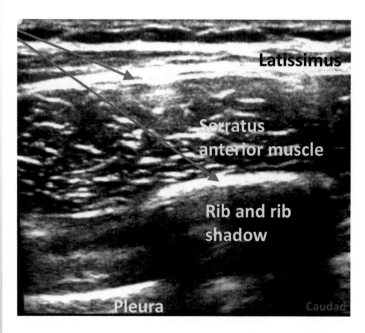

Fig. 2. Ultrasound image depicts the serratus anterior plane block. Orange arrows depict needle trajectory for both superficial and deep local anesthetic placement options.

In a small study versus TEA, SAP block was found to have comparable analgesia and reduced side effects (such as hypotension), in the early postoperative period.[41] In another study, VAS scores were compared between SAP block and PVB, revealing similar analgesia for the first 12 hours after thoracotomy; however, PVB was superior to SAP after 12 hours. There was no hypotension from SAP block, in contrast with 13% of the PVB group.[42] Another small study compared SAP block with TEA with no hypotension in the SAP block group; however, better VAS scores were reported in the epidural group after 12 hours.[43]

POST-THORACOTOMY PAIN SYNDROME

Chronic PTPS affects a large portion of patients undergoing thoracic surgery. It is estimated that almost 50% of patients have persistent pain at 6 months and even 20% may continue to experience pain at 6 to 7 years.[1,44] Patients complain of intermittent or constant burning, numbness, or a cutting sensation along the thoracotomy scar. Predictors of PTPS include those that increase acute pain, such as the previously mentioned patient factors and incision type, as well as the consumption of analgesics during the first postoperative week.[45] Perioperative TEA has been shown to decrease the incidence of PTPS; however, preemptive analgesia has not.

PTPS has a significant neuropathic component, making opioids less effective, which has led to rapid acceleration of dosing, without improvement. Pharmacologic agents that have been shown to improve PTPS include gabapentinoids, ketamine, tricyclic antidepressants, serotonin–norepinephrine reputable inhibitors, and lidocaine patches.[46] Regional anesthesia such as ESP blocks may improve PTPS as well.[2] The goal is to reduce the peripheral and central sensitization that has occurred by acting at the source of pain, as opposed to just dulling the discomfort centrally.

SUMMARY

When caring for a patient undergoing thoracic surgery, adequate pain management is a critical aspect of their recovery. A multimodal pharmacologic approach combined with regional anesthesia optimizes analgesia and minimizes adverse effects from opioids after thoracic surgery. The decision regarding which nerve block is most appropriate for the patient depends on the patient's medical history and comorbidities, and the physician's expertise.

A VATS approach has many advantages, but should involve some form of regional anesthesia. If a surgeon-placed ICNB is preferred, liposomal bupivacaine may be a superior option to plain local anesthetic, owing to an increased duration of the block. When converting from VATS or RATS to open thoracotomy, TEA or PVB should be considered postoperatively. If anticoagulation is an issue, ESP block is an alternative.

Thoracotomy necessitates regional anesthesia, if possible. TEA or PVB remain the gold standards. The choice between TEA and PVB should be at the discretion of the anesthesia team and their expertise. In the event that TEA and PVB are con-traindicated owing to anticoagulation, ICNB, ESP block, or SAP block should be used as a part of a multimodal analgesic plan.

When regional nerve blocks are contraindicated owing to disseminated bacteremia or diffuse cellu-litis, a multimodal pharmacologic approach should be used to minimize opioids. Ketamine may be an appropriate option in these scenarios. Considering the impact of opioid side effects and addiction po-tential on patients, there should be no role for opioid-only analgesia in the thoracic surgery pa-tient. Opioids may still be necessary; however, minimizing the prescribed dose should decrease tolerance and dependence.

DISCLOSURE

The authors have nothing to disclose.

REFERENCES

1. Kolettas A, Lazaridis G, Baka S, et al. Postoperative pain management. J Thorac Dis 2015;7(S1):S62–72.

2. Mesbah A, Yeung J, Gao F. Pain after thoracotomy. BJA Educ 2016;16:1–7.

3. Pennefather SH, McKevith J. Pain management after thoracic surgery. In: Slinger P, editor. Principles and practice of anesthesia for thoracic surgery. New York: Springer; 2011. p. 675–99.

4. Bennett GJ. Update on the neurophysiology of pain transmission and modulation: focus on the NMDA-receptor. J Pain Symptom Manage 2000;19(S1): S2–6.

5. Brescia AA, Harrington CA, Mazurek AA, et al. Fac-tors associated with new persistent opioid usage af-ter lung resection. Ann Thorac Surg 2019;107(2): 363–8.

6. Gottschalk A, Cohen SP, Yang S, et al. Preventing and treating pain after thoracic surgery. Anesthesi-ology 2006;104:594–600.

7. Veronesi G, Novellis P, Voulaz E, et al. Robot-assis-ted surgery for lung cancer: state of the art and per-spectives. Lung Cancer 2016;101:28–34.

8. Swanson SJ, Miller DL, Mckenna RJ, et al. Comparing robot-assisted thoracic surgical lobec-tomy with conventional video-assisted thoracic sur-gical lobectomy and wedge resection: results from a multihospital database (Premier). J Thorac Cardio-vasc Surg 2014;147(3):929–37.

9. Van der ploeg APT, Ayez N, Akkersdijk GP, et al. Postoperative pain after lobectomy: robot-assisted, video-assisted and open thoracic surgery. J Robot Surg 2020;14(1):131–6.

10. Agzarian J, Fahim C, Shargall Y, et al. The use of robotic-assisted thoracic surgery for lung resection: a comprehensive systematic review. Semin Thorac Cardiovasc Surg 2016;28(1):182–92.

11. Juan H. Prostaglandins as modulators of pain. Gen Pharmacol 1978;9(6):403–9.

12. Maxwell C, Nicoara A. New developments in the treatment of acute pain after thoracic surgery. Curr Opin Anaesthesiol 2014;27(1):6–11.

13. Whelton A. Nephrotoxicity of nonsteroidal anti-inflammatory drugs: physiologic foundations and clinical implications. Am J Med 1999;106(5B): 13S–24S.

14. Chumbley GM, Thompson L, Swatman JE, et al. Ke-tamine infusion for 96 hr after thoracotomy: effects on acute and persistent pain. Eur J Pain 2019; 23(5):985–93.

15. Mathews TJ, Churchhouse AM, Housden T, et al. Does adding ketamine to morphine patient-controlled analgesia safely improve post-thoracotomy pain? Interact Cardiovasc Thorac Surg 2012;14(2):194–9.

16. Nesher N, Serovian I, Marouani N, et al. Ketamine spares morphine consumption after transthoracic lung and heart surgery without adverse hemody-namic effects. Pharmacol Res 2008;58(1):38–44.

17. Moyse DW, Kaye AD, Diaz JH, et al. Perioperative ketamine administration for thoracotomy pain. Pain Physician 2017;20(3):173–84.

18. Graham GG, Scott KF. Mechanism of action of para-cetamol. Am J Ther 2005;12(1):46–55.

19. Remy C, Marret E, Bonnet F. Effects of acetamino-phen on morphine side-effects and consumption af-ter major surgery: meta-analysis of randomized controlled trials. Br J Anaesth 2005;94(4):505–13.

20. Yoon E, Babar A, Choudhary M, et al. Acetamino-phen-induced hepatotoxicity: a comprehensive up-date. J Clin Transl Hepatol 2016;4(2):131–42.

21. Yu Y, Liu N, Zeng Q, et al. The efficacy of pregabalin for the management of acute and chronic postoper-ative pain in thoracotomy: a meta-analysis with trial sequential analysis of randomized-controlled trials. J Pain Res 2019;12:159–70.

22. Adams JM, Giroir BP. Opioid prescribing trends and the physician's role in responding to the public health crisis. JAMA Intern Med 2019;179(4):476–8.

23. Kissin I. Preemptive analgesia. Anesthesiology 2000;93(4):1138–43.

24. Bong CL, Samuel M, Ng JM, et al. Effects of pre-emptive epidural analgesia on post-thoracotomy pain. J Cardiothorac Vasc Anesth 2005;19(6): 786–93.

25. Møiniche S, Kehlet H, Dahl JB. A qualitative and quantitative systematic review of preemptive anal-gesia for postoperative pain relief: the role of timing of analgesia. Anesthesiology 2002;96(3):725–41.

26. Horlocker TT, Vandermeulen E, Kopp SL, et al. Regional anesthesia in the patient receiving antith-rombotic or thrombolytic therapy: American Society

of Regional Anesthesia and Pain Medicine Evidence-Based Guidelines (Fourth Edition). Reg Anesth Pain Med 2018;43(3):263–309.

27. Yeung JH, Gates S, Naidu BV, et al. Paravertebral block versus thoracic epidural for patients undergoing thoracotomy. Cochrane Database Syst Rev 2016;(2):CD009121.

28. Biswas S, Verma R, Bhatia VK, et al. Comparison between thoracic epidural block and thoracic paravertebral block for post thoracotomy pain relief. J Clin Diagn Res 2016;10(9):UC08–12.

29. Tamura T, Mori S, Mori A, et al. A randomized controlled trial comparing paravertebral block via the surgical field with thoracic epidural block using ropivacaine for post-thoracotomy pain relief. J Anesth 2017;31(2):263–70.

30. Wurnig PN, Lackner H, Teiner C, et al. Is intercostal block for pain management in thoracic surgery more successful than epidural anaesthesia? Eur J Cardiothorac Surg 2002;21(6):1115–9.

31. Bousema JE, Dias EM, Hagen SM, et al. Subpleural multilevel intercostal continuous analgesia after thoracoscopic pulmonary resection: a pilot study. J Cardiothorac Surg 2019;14(1):179.

32. Khalil KG, Boutrous ML, Irani AD, et al. Operative intercostal nerve blocks with long-acting bupivacaine liposome for pain control after thoracotomy. Ann Thorac Surg 2015;100(6):2013–8.

33. Rice DC, Cata JP, Mena GE, et al. Posterior intercostal nerve block with liposomal bupivacaine: an alternative to thoracic epidural analgesia. Ann Thorac Surg 2015;99(6):1953–60.

34. Pitre L, Garbee D, Tipton J, et al. Effects of preoperative intrathecal morphine on postoperative intravenous morphine dosage: a systematic review protocol. JBI Database System Rev Implement Rep 2018;16(4):867–70.

35. Chin KJ. Thoracic wall blocks: from paravertebral to retrolaminar to serratus to erector spinae and back again - A review of evidence. Best Pract Res Clin Anaesthesiol 2019;33(1):67–77.

36. Fang B, Wang Z, Huang X. Ultrasound-guided preoperative single-dose erector spinae plane block provides comparable analgesia to thoracic

paravertebral block following thoracotomy: a single center randomized controlled double-blind study. Ann Transl Med 2019;7(8):174.

37. Adhikary SD, Prasad A, Soleimani B, et al. Continuous erector spinae plane block as an effective analgesic option in anticoagulated patients after left ventricular assist device implantation: a case series. J Cardiothorac Vasc Anesth 2019;33(4):1063–7.

38. Luis-navarro JC, Seda-guzmán M, Luis-moreno C, et al. The erector spinae plane block in 4 cases of video-assisted thoracic surgery. Rev Esp Anestesiol Reanim 2018;65(4):204–8.

39. Forero M, Rajarathinam M, Adhikary S, et al. Erector spinae plane (ESP) block in the management of post thoracotomy pain syndrome: a case series. Scand J Pain 2017;17:325–9.

40. Semyonov M, Fedorina E, Grinshpun J, et al. Ultrasound-guided serratus anterior plane block for analgesia after thoracic surgery. J Pain Res 2019;12:953–60.

41. Ökmen K, Ökmen BM. The efficacy of serratus anterior plane block in analgesia for thoracotomy: a retrospective study. J Anesth 2017;31(4):579–85.

42. Saad FS, El Baradie SY, Abdel Aliem MAW, et al. Ultrasound-guided serratus anterior plane block versus thoracic paravertebral block for perioperative analgesia in thoracotomy. Saudi J Anaesth 2018;12(4):565–70.

43. Khalil AE, Abdallah NM, Bashandy GM, et al. Ultrasound-guided serratus anterior plane block versus thoracic epidural analgesia for thoracotomy pain. J Cardiothorac Vasc Anesth 2017;31(1):152–8.

44. Bayman EO, Brennan TJ. Incidence and severity of chronic pain at 3 and 6 months after thoracotomy: meta-analysis. J Pain 2014;15(9):887–97.

45. Blichfeldt-eckhardt MR, Andersen C, Ørding H, et al. From acute to chronic pain after thoracic surgery: the significance of different components of the acute pain response. J Pain Res 2018;11:1541–8.

46. Dworkin RH, O'connor AB, Audette J, et al. Recommendations for the pharmacological management of neuropathic pain: an overview and literature update. Mayo Clin Proc 2010;85(3 Suppl):S3–14.

Management of Complications After Lung Resection
Prolonged Air Leak and Bronchopleural Fistula

James M. Clark, MD, David T. Cooke, MD, Lisa M. Brown, MD, MAS*

KEYWORDS

- Bronchopleural fistula • Air leak • Thoracic surgery • Perioperative management

KEY POINTS

- Prolonged air leak or bronchoalveolar fistula is common and can usually be managed with continued pleural drainage until resolution.
- Bronchopleural fistula is rare but is associated with high mortality, often caused by development of concomitant empyema.
- Bronchopleural fistula should be confirmed with bronchoscopy and often can be treated endoscopically, but may require operative stump revision or window thoracostomy.

PROLONGED AIR LEAK
Background

The most common postoperative complication after elective lung resection is an alveolar-pleural fistula, or air leak.[1] An air leak is defined as a communication between the alveoli of the pulmonary parenchyma distal to a segmental bronchus with the pleural space.[2,3] Prolonged air leak (PAL) is defined by the Society of Thoracic Surgeons (STS) General Thoracic Surgery Database (GTSD) as an air leak persisting longer than 5 days postoperatively. The incidence of air leak after lung resection is 25% to 50% on postoperative day 1 and up to 20% on day 2.[4,5] Although most air leaks resolve spontaneously with chest tube drainage, the incidence of PAL after lung cancer resection was 10% over the past decade within the STS GTSD,[6] and 15% to 25% in other reports.[7,8]

PAL negatively affects other perioperative outcomes. Patients with PAL have significantly increased length of stay, leading to increased cost. Among nonpneumonectomy lung resection patients, those with PAL, compared with those without, had a mean length of stay of 7.2 versus 4.8 days (*P*<.001) and a 30% increase in the inpatient costs ($26,070 vs $19,558; *P*<.001).[9] Similar results were shown in a cohort of video-assisted thoracoscopic surgery (VATS) lung cancer resection patients, with mean length of stay nearly twice as long compared with those without a PAL (11.7 vs 6.5 days; *P*<.001).[10] These results are corroborated in the National Emphysema Treatment Trial data (11.8 vs 7.6 days; *P*<.001).[11] Medicare patients with PAL for 7 to 10 days after lung resection and greater than 10 days after lung resection had 30% and 100%, respectively, greater inpatient hospital costs compared with those with PAL less than 7 days (*P*<.001).[12] Postoperative intensive care unit readmission rates may be higher with PAL (9% vs 5%; *P* = .05),[13] likely caused by associated complications such as pneumonia and empyema.[11,14] The incidence of empyema is 10.4% with PAL greater than 7 days, compared with 1% with air leaks less than or equal to

Section of General Thoracic Surgery, Department of Surgery, University of California, Davis Health, 2335 Stockton Boulevard, 6th Floor North Addition Office Building, Sacramento, CA 95817, USA
* Corresponding author.
E-mail address: lmbrown@ucdavis.edu
Twitter: @JamesClarkMD (J.M.C.); @DavidCookeMD (D.T.C.); @LisaBrownMD (L.M.B.)

Thorac Surg Clin 30 (2020) 347–358
https://doi.org/10.1016/j.thorsurg.2020.04.008
1547-4127/20/© 2020 Elsevier Inc. All rights reserved.

7 days (P = .01).[15] PAL requires prolonged chest tube drainage, which increases postoperative pain,[1,16] respiratory splinting leading to increased pneumonia risk,[11] venous thromboembolic risk caused by diminished mobility,[16] and necessity for additional procedures such as chemical or mechanical pleurodesis.[17] In addition, the PAL rate was twice as high among readmitted lobectomy patients compared with those who did not require readmission (21.4% vs 10.2%; $P<.001$).[18] PAL also is associated with increased in-hospital mortality.[13] Patients with an air leak have a 3.4 times greater risk of death than those without (95% confidence interval [CI], 1.9–6.2).[9]

PREOPERATIVE RISK FACTORS
Demographic Factors

Patients undergoing lung resection who develop PAL are often older than those who do not,[19] with many PAL predictive tools using an age cutoff of greater than 65 years.[20] Men are 11% to 39% more likely than women to have a PAL.[6,9]

Clinical Factors

Patients with a lower body mass index are at increased risk of PAL, with cutoff less than or equal to 25 kg/m^2 commonly studied.[6,20] Emphysematous disease processes such as chronic obstructive pulmonary disease dramatically increase the odds of PAL.[9] Resection through emphysematous bullous tissue can make adequate sealing of parenchymal transection lines with staplers more challenging. Decreased forced expiratory volume in 1 second (FEV$_1$) is a strong independent predictor for PAL.[6,11,20,21] Lower diffusion capacity of the lung for carbon monoxide (DLCO) also increases the risk of PAL.[11,20] Several case series of patients with pulmonary disease associated with infectious agents such as tuberculosis and aspergillosis have shown a high risk of PAL.[22–24]

INTRAOPERATIVE RISK FACTORS

Larger parenchymal resections tend to increase the risk of PAL. Fissure dissection during lobectomy and bilobectomy, particularly in the setting of an incomplete fissure, can cause parenchymal tears leading to air leaks.[1,25] Using a fissureless dissection technique significantly reduces the risk of PAL (odds ratio [OR], 0.32; 95% CI, 0.22–0.51).[25] In addition, longer staple lines required for lobectomies rather than sublobar resections increase the length over which a staple line air leak can potentially occur. As such, lobectomy has been shown to have 1.5 to 2.0 times increased odds of PAL compared with segmentectomy or wedge resection.[9,13] When comparing types of lobar resections, resection of upper lobes regardless of laterality has been shown to increase the odds of PAL.[13] Concordantly, review of the Cleveland Clinic experience in lobectomies found that resection of the left lower lobe was an independent predictor for protection against PAL.[26]

Presence of pleural adhesions, which can be highly vascular and require extensive adhesiolysis, is a substantial risk factor for PAL.[11] Pleural adhesions were the only independent risk factor for PAL in a recent cohort of 1051 lung cancer resection patients (OR, 2.38; 95% CI, 1.43–3.95)[10] and are an important intraoperative risk factor in several PAL prediction scores.[20,27,28]

POSTOPERATIVE RISK FACTORS

Postoperative mechanical ventilation is the only postoperative risk factor identified for development of PAL,[29] with up to a 19% incidence of air leak in pneumonectomy patients requiring postoperative ventilation.[30]

PROLONGED AIR LEAK PREDICTIVE SCORES

Numerous investigators have proposed scoring systems to predict the risk of PAL.[6,20,27,28,31–36] Brunelli and colleagues[32] proposed a PAL risk score in 2004 including FEV$_1$, pleural adhesions, and upper lobe resections.[20] Their group revised and validated their score in 2010, based on 4 factors: age greater than 65 years (1 point), pleural adhesions (1 point), FEV$_1$ less than 80% (1.5 points), and body mass index (BMI) less than 25.5 kg/m^2 (2 points) (**Table 1**). PAL risk increased stepwise with each class: class A (0 points), 1.4%; class B (1 point), 5.0%; class C (1.5–3 points), 12.5%; class D (>3 points), 29.0%. Lee and colleagues[27] devised a PAL prediction tool based on the Canadian experience that similarly included pleural adhesions, FEV$_1$, and DLCO, and a more complex index of PAL model was produced by French investigators including male sex, BMI, dyspnea score, pleural

Table 1 Aggregate prolonged air leak risk score derived by Brunelli and colleagues[32]	
	Points
Age >65 y	1
Presence of pleural adhesions	1
Forced expiratory volume in 1 s <80%	1.5
BMI<25.5 kg/m^2	2

From Brunelli A, Varela G, Refai M, et al. A scoring system to predict the risk of prolonged air leak after lobectomy. Ann Thorac Surg. 2010;90(1):206; with permission.

adhesions, lobectomy or segmentectomy, bilobectomy, bullae resection, pulmonary volume reduction, and upper lobe resection.[28,34] Brunelli and colleagues[33] have updated their own European Society of Thoracic Surgeons risk score, finding that male gender, FEV_1 less than 80%, and BMI less than or equal to 18.5 kg/m^2 better predict PAL in VATS patients.

An STS GTSD study of 52,198 patients formulated a PAL score dichotomizing patients as either high or low risk. The score includes all variables easily determined preoperatively: BMI less than or equal to 25 kg/m^2 (7 points), lobectomy or bilobectomy (6 points), FEV_1 less than or equal to 70% (5 points), male sex (4 points), and right upper lobe (3 points) (**Table 2**). A score greater than 17 points predicted a high PAL risk compared with less than or equal to 17 points as a low PAL risk (19.6 vs 9% incidence, respectively), with a sensitivity of 30%, specificity of 85%, negative predictive value of 91%, and positive predictive value of 19%.

AIR LEAK EVALUATION

An air leak is identified by observing air bubbling into the water seal chamber of the pleural drainage canister. Such a finding warns that removal of a chest tube is likely to result in continued parenchymal air leak with subsequent pneumothorax development. Recently, digital drainage systems have been developed to better objectively evaluate air leaks.[37] Such drainage systems can provide real-time monitoring of continuous air flow and pleural pressure as well as accurate drainage volume measurements.[38] A recent Japanese study found that persistent air flow greater than or equal to 20 mL/min at 36 hours postoperatively was highly predictive of PAL, with sensitivity and specificity of 91% and 73%, respectively, and receiver operating characteristic c-statistic of 0.88 (95% CI, 0.80–0.96).[39] A Canadian group used modeling of

Table 2	
Prolonged air leak score derived by Seder and colleagues[6]	
	Points
BMI $\leq$ 25 kg/m^2	7
Lobectomy or bilobectomy	6
Forced expiratory volume in 1 s $\leq$70%	5
Male sex	4
Right upper lobe procedure	3

From Seder CW, Basu S, Ramsay T, et al. A prolonged air leak score for lung cancer resection: an analysis of the STS GTSD. Ann Thorac Surg. 2019;108(5):1480; with permission.

digital drainage system data to accurately predict air leak recurrence after chest tube removal with sensitivity of 80% and specificity of 88%.[40] Other studies have found no difference in chest tube duration or length of stay with the use of digital drainage systems.[5] Although widespread implementation of digital pleural drainage systems to improve chest tube removal decision making has been slow to gain traction, this may change in the future as health systems attempt to identify ways to reduce prolonged lengths of stay.

PRINCIPLES OF MANAGEMENT

Most uncomplicated alveolar-pleural fistulae resolve with chest tube drainage and expectant management.[41] Although chest tube management strategies vary, many surgeons advocate keeping chest tubes on −20 cm of water suction until the morning of postoperative day 1, at which time tubes are transitioned to water seal.[4,42,43] A small air leak at this time may be best managed on water seal, but a new or enlarging pneumothorax or development of subcutaneous emphysema should prompt return to suction.[44] A meta-analysis of 7 randomized trials found no differences in the incidence of PAL, chest tube duration, or hospital stay when comparing initial postoperative chest tube management on suction versus water seal.[45]

With the advent of portable pleural drainage systems, outpatient management of PAL is feasible and common, given that most resolve with adequate visceral and parietal pleural apposition.[46] Thus, patients can be safely discharged with chest tube in place for outpatient leak testing and removal.[47,48] Such strategies may in part contribute to increasing postoperative day 1 discharges after anatomic lung resections, without increased risk of mortality or readmission.[49–51] Four percent of STS GTSD contributing centers discharge more than 20% of anatomic lung resection patients on postoperative day 1.[50] However, this must be balanced with recent data indicating a 25% readmission rate and nearly 17% incidence of empyema in patients discharged with a chest tube after pulmonary resection, with more than 12% requiring decortication.[52]

More aggressive management strategies have been explored for PAL, such as chemical pleurodesis (with tetracycline, talc, iodine, or silver nitrate),[17,53] blood patch administration,[54] and endobronchial 1-way valve placement,[55–58] which have shown some efficacy. None of these techniques have been compared in a randomized fashion, but case series have shown PAL resolution rates of greater than 95% with chemical pleurodesis, greater than 92% with autologous blood patches, and greater than 93% with endobronchial valve (EBV) placement.[17]

BRONCHOPLEURAL FISTULA
Background

In contrast with alveolar-pleural fistulae, a bronchopleural fistula (BPF) is defined as a communication between a main stem, lobar, or sublobar bronchus with the pleural space.[59] The incidence of BPF is less than or equal to 1% for lobectomy and sublobar resections and 4% to 20% after pneumonectomy.[60–62]

Historically, the mortality associated with BPF ranged from 20% to 50%.[60,63–67] Modern series show a mortality of 11% to 18% for early BPF (within 30 days of surgery)[62,68,69] and 0% to 7% for late BPF (beyond 30 days of surgery).[68–70] BPF mortality risk is particularly high after pneumonectomy because there is often concomitant empyema caused by failure to control the bronchial stump leak, resulting in pneumonia of the remaining contralateral lung. Empyema after lobectomy likely occurs as a combination of PAL, percutaneous drain as a potential infectious nidus, and persistent pleural space.[71] In contrast, more than 75% of postpneumonectomy empyemas occur in the setting of a bronchial stump BPF.[62,72,73] The cause of BPF-induced empyema is direct pleural space contamination by mucocutaneous, respiratory, or digestive tract microbes. BPF-associated empyema carries a significant risk of cardiopulmonary complications, in excess of 61.5% versus 11.4% in patients without BPF (P<.001), and a mortality risk of 30.8% versus 3.9% in patients without BPF (P<.001).[29] BPF in conjunction with postpneumonectomy empyema has repeatedly been shown to be an independent predictor of mortality,[67,74] especially early in the postoperative course when mortality ranges from 11.6% to 18% compared with late BPF from 0% to 7.1%.[68,69] More recent data from France reported early (within 2 weeks of surgery) BPF-associated empyema mortalities of 19% compared with 5% when empyema occurs later (after postoperative day 14).[63] Survival differences become even more pronounced over time, with 1-year survival of 80% versus 47% for late versus early postpneumonectomy empyema (P = .01).[63] As such, this complication, which is primarily seen in pneumonectomy patients, must be recognized and addressed early to prevent significant morbidity and mortality.

PREOPERATIVE RISK FACTORS
Demographic Factors

Similar to alveolar-pleura fistulae, advanced age increases the risk of BPF. Age cutoffs of greater than 60 years and greater than 70 years have been shown to dramatically increase the risk of BPF development, with ORs of 1.18 (95% CI, 1.12–1.62) to 2.14 (95% CI, 1.14–3.93), respectively.[68,69] A recent French BPF prediction model found that men had a 2.63 times greater odds of postpneumonectomy BPF than women (P<.001).[75]

Clinical Factors

Diabetic microangiopathy causes small vessel ischemia throughout the end organs of the body, and the bronchial stump circulation is particularly prone to poor wound healing secondary to ischemia.[71,76] A recent meta-analysis found that diabetic patients undergoing pulmonary resection had pooled increased odds of BPF of 1.97 (95% CI, 1.39–2.80) compared with nondiabetic patients,[77] which is corroborated in other BPF risk models.[68] Preoperative albumin level less than 3.5 g/dL is an independent predictor of BPF after pneumonectomy (P = .02), suggesting that poor wound healing of the bronchial stump leads to BPF development.[78] In addition, low BMI has been shown to increase BPF risk, with each additional 1-kg/m^2 decrease in BMI increasing the odds of BPF by 1.7 times (P<.001).[75]

Benign Lung Disease

In general, the risk of BPF after pneumonectomy is higher for benign pulmonary disease, primarily infectious, rather than for cancer resections. Most case series analyzing BPF describe patients undergoing completion pneumonectomy (during which the risk of operative complications is invariably higher), because primary pneumonectomy for benign disease is rare.[79–84] Analysis of the STS GTSD pneumonectomy experience shows 2.8 times greater odds of major complication, including empyema and BPF, for patients with benign disease versus lung cancer (95% CI, 1.35–5.82).[85] The French experience found that, of 5975 pneumonectomies over a decade, only 3.4% and 2.0% underwent pneumonectomy and completion pneumonectomy, respectively, for benign conditions.[86] However, these patients had a significantly higher complication rate (53% vs 39%) and in-hospital mortality (22% vs 5%) compared with those undergoing pneumonectomy for malignancy (P<.001). Other factors contribute to this increased risk of BPF and mortality in pneumonectomy patients with benign pathology. Thirty-seven percent of the pneumonectomies for benign disease were done in a nonelective fashion (compared with only 1.6% for malignant disease), which is a known risk factor for operative complications. In addition, pulmonary decortications and resections for infectious disease are fraught with complication risk caused by dense adhesions and an infected operative field.[71,87] Highly vascularized adhesions can cause significant bleeding and also increase the risk of bronchial ischemia intraoperatively. In addition, the proinflammatory state of acute infections such as pneumonia has been shown to increase the risk of BPF.[69,88]

Neoadjuvant Therapy

For patients with malignancy, there are mixed results on the risk of BPF associated with induction chemotherapy. One purported effect is the risk of poor wound healing associated with chemotherapy.[80] One study from MD Anderson reported zero incidence of BPF or empyema in lobectomy and pneumonectomy patients who received neoadjuvant chemotherapy.[89] This finding was corroborated by more recent data from Pittsburgh, where investigators found similar BPF and empyema rates between patients receiving neoadjuvant chemotherapy versus upfront pneumonectomy (8.8% vs 7.3%; P = .61). Analysis by Hu and colleagues[68] of 684 patients undergoing pneumonectomy found neoadjuvant therapy to be an independent predictor of BPF (hazard ratio, 2.48; 95% CI, 0.05–0.28).

To this end, a recent meta-analysis of 30 studies of 14,912 lung cancer resection patients found that neoadjuvant chemotherapy alone did not increase the risk of BPF (OR, 1.86; 95% CI, 0.88–3.91).[90] Neoadjuvant radiotherapy alone (OR, 3.91; 95% CI, 1.40–10.94) or as combination chemoradiotherapy (OR, 2.53; 95% CI, 1.35–4.74) significantly increased the risk of BPF. Similarly, neoadjuvant radiotherapy was an independent predictor of late (but not early) BPF in the Shanghai experience (OR, 2.83; 95% CI, 3.12–30.96).[68] Radiotherapy induces bronchial mucosa ischemia,[91] but the mucosal blood flow can recover in as little as 8 to 10 days after completion of therapy.[92] Early radiation can cause mucosal edema and inhibit capillary angiogenesis, but late effects can cause fibrotic small vessel disease through radiation vasculopathy.[91] In addition, radiation-induced mucosal ischemia may be exacerbated by the ischemia from bronchial vessel disruption associated with lymphadenectomy during lung cancer resection.[71]

POSTOPERATIVE RISK FACTORS

Immediate or early extubation should be the goal because prolonged positive pressure ventilation is an independent risk factor for early BPF.[29] The incidence of BPF can be as high as 19% in patients requiring mechanical ventilation postoperatively.[30,61]

DIAGNOSIS

The signs and symptoms of BPF after lung resection can be varied and nonspecific, therefore it is important to have a high index of suspicion. Signs of empyema (leukocytosis, fever, pleural fluid on imaging, and purulence fluid on thoracentesis) should raise the concern for an underlying BPF. Continued air leak is common after lung resection, but a large continuous air leak should immediately raise the suspicion for air leaking from a bronchial rather than a parenchymal source. Development of a pneumothorax after chest tube removal could represent a continued parenchymal PAL, but a large pneumothorax days or weeks after resection is highly concerning for a BPF.

The classic radiographic sign of postpneumonectomy BPF is a decreasing air-fluid level over time (≥2 cm), indicating displacement of the postoperative pleural fluid (**Fig. 1**). During this time, the patient often has a persistent and worsening cough, and is at risk of developing pneumonia in the contralateral lung.[71] All patients suspected of having a BPF should be evaluated with a chest computed tomography scan and flexible bronchoscopy. Saline can be instilled during bronchoscopy to look for bubbling at the staple line. If radiographic and bronchoscopic findings are still equivocal, transthoracic exploration and submersion of the stump under saline for a bubble test under positive pressure ventilation can make the definitive diagnosis.

PRINCIPLES OF MANAGEMENT

If empyema is suspected or confirmed, antibiotics are necessary. Most BPF-associated empyema is monomicrobial, with the most common pathogens being *Staphylococcus* and *Streptococcus* species.[63] Next, adequate drainage should be established by placement of a thoracostomy tube and instillation of fibrinolytics if the empyema is loculated.[78]

In postpneumonectomy BPF, care should be taken to avoid spillage of any empyema into the contralateral lung by keeping the patient upright at least at 45° and decubitus on the operative side down if able.[71] After drainage of the pleural space, bronchoscopy should be used to identify the BPF and to assess the viability and length of the bronchial stump. As discussed earlier, thoracoscopy can be paired with bronchoscopy to identify occult BPFs with a saline leak test under positive pressure.

In appropriately selected patients, BPF can be treated via endobronchial therapy, avoiding a major reoperation. Small defects (<5 mm) in patients

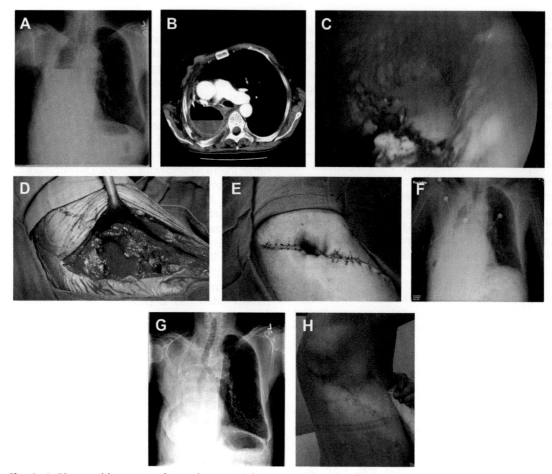

Fig. 1. A 59-year-old woman who underwent right pneumonectomy for adenocarcinoma and 16 years later developed failure to thrive secondary to chronic postpneumonectomy empyema. Chest radiograph at presentation with air-fluid level (*A*). Computed tomography imaging showing BPF and empyema (*B*). Empyema intraoperatively (*C*) during bronchial stump closure with Eloesser thoracostomy window intraoperative dissection (*D*) and creation (*E*). She then underwent omental flap and partial chest wall closure with a pleural drainage system 8 weeks after Eloesser thoracostomy window, as seen on chest radiograph (*F*). She eventually had the drainage system removed with resolution of the BPF and empyema on chest radiograph (*G*), and chest wall wound closure with latissimus dorsi flap coverage 18 weeks after initial Eloesser thoracostomy window creation (*H*).

without sepsis can often be managed with endoscopic fibrin glue[93,94] or silver nitrate.[64,95] Fibrin glue can have high rates of success, up to 100% after 2 to 3 applications.[94] Silver nitrate has been shown to have success rates ranging from 80% to 100%.[64,95] A Japanese case series of 7 patients showed 100% success with bronchoscopic instillation of a polyglycolic acid mesh with fibrin glue over the fistula area.[96] Most recently, airway stenting has shown considerable success, with 97% first-attempt and 100% second-attempt success rates in a series of 148 patients from China.[97]

Nevertheless, the need for operative reexploration is common, with historical case series indicating rates of greater than 90% and reclosure of the bronchial stump in nearly half of those cases.[61] The need for and success of reoperative

interventions depend on many factors, including early versus late presentation, dehiscence size, length of the bronchial stump, quality of the remnant stump tissue, presence of remnant malignancy at the stump site, and extent of contamination of the ipsilateral pleural cavity or infectious involvement of the contralateral lung.[30] In general, early dehiscence tends to be more amenable to immediate repair or stump revision, whereas late dehiscence can be more technically challenging to repair because of diminished tissue quality, development of a matured fistula tract, and significant pleural contamination and scarring.[71] Longer stumps should be trimmed back to healthier tissue leaving a minimum of 3 mm of remnant bronchial stump length,[98] and, if there is insufficient length for a new staple line, then direct suture repair

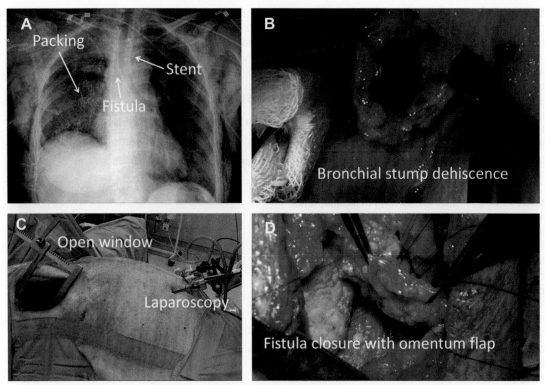

Fig. 2. Repair of a BPF in a staged fashion starting with placement of a conical stent to exclude the fistula from airflow (*A*), open thoracotomy pleural washout and packing with antibiotic-soaked gauzes (*B*), followed by laparoscopic omental harvesting (*C*) and BPF primary closure buttressed with an omental flap (*D*). (*From* Andreetti C, Menna C, D'Andrilli A, et al. Multimodal treatment for post-pneumonectomy bronchopleural fistula associated with empyema. Ann Thorac Surg. 2018;106(6):e338; with permission.)

should be performed with absorbable, monofilament, pledgeted sutures with vascularized tissue buttressing.[71] Dehiscence of greater than 50% of the bronchial stump is associated with dramatically delayed time to successful stump closure.[99] A recent South Korean case suggests empiric musculocutaneous flap coverage of any BPF with dehiscence of 1 cm or greater.[100] Repair of a late dehiscence is often impractical because extensive dissection of the stump can be risky. Tissue transfers into the pleural cavity (muscle or omental flaps) can cover the bronchial stump and eliminate the persistent pleural space (**Fig. 2**).

In patients are unable to tolerate bronchial stump revision or if early repair fails, open window thoracostomy (OWT) should be considered because adequate drainage allows most fistulae to close over time. An OWT, such as the Eloesser flap, is created by removal of a portion of 2 or 3 ribs at the most dependent portion of the empyema cavity with marsupialization of the subcutaneous tissues/skin flaps to the pleura, with success rates as high as 60% to 90%[22,101,102] (see **Fig. 1**). The original Eloesser flap was expanded to a 2-stage Clagett procedure

wherein, after adequate drainage, serial operative debridements, and local wound care, intrapleural antibiotic solution is instilled with definitive chest wall closure.[103] Obliteration of the pleural cavity can also be aided with muscular or omental flap transposition. Almost any nearby vascularized tissue pedicle can be used for buttressing, but common options include muscle flaps (latissimus dorsi, serratus anterior, intercostal),[104] parietal pleura,[105] pericardium,[106] pericardial fat,[107] pericardiophrenic graft,[107] azygos vein on the right side,[105] rectus abdominis myocutaneous flaps,[108] and omentum,[109,110] which can be harvested from a thoracotomy through a transdiaphragmatic approach.[111]

The duration of OWT is patient dependent and depends on response to antibiotic therapy, obliteration of the empyema cavity, nutrition status, and strict adherence to tobacco cessation efforts.[98] A recent Italian case series had a median duration of OWT of 5 months (range, 3–9 months) and found that early OWT creation increased the success of BPF healing.[101] Despite these encouraging results, other contemporary case series report dismal long-term survival after OWT of only 8%

at 4 years,[78] and ongoing packing of an open thoracic wound is often poorly tolerated by patients.[112]

Recently, OWT has been paired with vacuum-assisted closure devices to improve patient tolerance of wound care and healing time.[113] In addition, the recent Swiss experience has shown success in reducing mean time to OWT closure to 8 days using a modified Clagett process with povidone-iodine–soaked sponge packing changed in the operating room every 48 hours to allow for serial debridements, leading to a 100% OWT closure success rate with 0% 3-month mortality.[66] For BPF after partial lung resection, a last resort can be completion lobectomy or bilobectomy to ensure bronchial stump closure at a level of the bronchial tree with healthy tissue. Main bronchial stump revision sometimes is best accomplished through a transsternal transpericardial approach to the carina, especially for left-sided and long-stump BPFs. This approach provides an uninfected and noninflamed operative field.[114] More recent case series have shown considerable success in managing BPF with thoracoscopic debridement and stump revision, obviating OWT in many patients.[70,115,116]

Evidence on the benefit of EBV placement in aiding BPF closure is emerging, although the data are limited to small case series. These 1-way valves limit airflow into the pleural space while allowing backflow of mucus and air.[117] EBV placement is most commonly used for persistent pneumothorax secondary to PAL as opposed to BPF with concomitant empyema; however, use in BPF is gaining traction.[118] One series of 3 critically ill mechanically ventilated patients with BPF found immediate air leak resolution after EBV placement followed by BPF resolution and extubation within 5 to 13 days and good long-term survival.[119] Other case reports have shown recovery from BPF in patients on extracorporeal membrane oxygenation[120] as well as in severe cystic fibrosis as a bridge to lung transplant.[121]

SUMMARY

PAL is common after lung resection but is usually managed with continued pleural drainage until resolution. Additional management options include blood patch administration, chemical pleurodesis, and 1-way EBV placement. BPF is rarer but significant because it is associated with a high mortality caused by development of concomitant empyema. BPF should be confirmed with bronchoscopy, which may allow bronchoscopic intervention. However, early operative intervention, especially when diagnosed early, with transthoracic stump revision or OWT may ultimately expedite BPF closure and improve survival.

DISCLOSURE

The authors have nothing to disclose.

REFERENCES

1. Mueller MR, Marzluf BA. The anticipation and management of air leaks and residual spaces post lung resection. J Thorac Dis 2014;6(3):271–84.
2. Kozower BD. 42 - Complications of thoracic surgical procedures. In: LoCicero J, Feins RH, Colson YL, et al, editors. Shields' general thoracic surgery. 8th edition. Philadelphia: Lippincott Williams & Wilkins; 2019. p. 573–85.
3. Cerfolio RJ. Advances in thoracostomy tube management. Surg Clin North Am 2002;82(4): 833–48, vii.
4. Cerfolio RJ, Bass C, Katholi CR. Prospective randomized trial compares suction versus water seal for air leaks. Ann Thorac Surg 2001;71(5):1613–7.
5. Gilbert S, McGuire AL, Maghera S, et al. Randomized trial of digital versus analog pleural drainage in patients with or without a pulmonary air leak after lung resection. J Thorac Cardiovasc Surg 2015; 150(5):1243–51.
6. Seder CW, Basu S, Ramsay T, et al. A prolonged air leak score for lung cancer resection: an analysis of the STS GTSD. Ann Thorac Surg 2019;108(5): 1478–83.
7. Cerfolio RJ, Pickens A, Bass C, et al. Fast-tracking pulmonary resections. J Thorac Cardiovasc Surg 2001;122(2):318–24.
8. Abolhoda A, Liu D, Brooks A, et al. Prolonged air leak following radical upper lobectomy: An analysis of incidence and possible risk factors. Chest 1998; 113(6):1507–10.
9. Yoo A, Ghosh SK, Danker W, et al. Burden of air leak complications in thoracic surgery estimated using a national hospital billing database. Clinicoecon Outcomes Res 2017;9:373–83.
10. Zhao K, Mei J, Xia C, et al. Prolonged air leak after video-assisted thoracic surgery lung cancer resection: Risk factors and its effect on postoperative clinical recovery. J Thorac Dis 2017;9(5):1219–25.
11. DeCamp MM, Blackstone EH, Naunheim KS, et al. Patient and surgical factors influencing air leak after lung volume reduction surgery: lessons learned from the national emphysema treatment trial. Ann Thorac Surg 2006;82(1):197–206.
12. Wood D, Lauer L, Layton A, et al. Prolonged length of stay associated with air leak following pulmonary

resection has a negative impact on hospital margin. Clinicoecon Outcomes Res 2016.

13. Elsayed H, McShane J, Shackcloth M. Air leaks following pulmonary resection for lung cancer: Is it a patient or surgeon related problem? Ann R Coll Surg Engl 2012.

14. Varela G, Jiménez MF, Novoa N, et al. Estimating hospital costs attributable to prolonged air leak in pulmonary lobectomy. Eur J Cardiothoracic Surg 2005.

15. Brunelli A, Xiume F, Al Refai M, et al. Air leaks after lobectomy increase the risk of empyema but not of cardiopulmonary complications: A case-matched analysis. Chest 2006.

16. Sánchez PG, Vendrame GS, Madke GR, et al. Lobectomy for treating bronchial carcinoma: Analysis of comorbidities and their impact on postoperative morbidity and mortality. J Bras Pneumol 2006.

17. Dugan KC, Laxmanan B, Murgu S, et al. Management of persistent air leaks. Chest 2017.

18. Brown LM, Thibault DP, Kosinski AS, et al. Readmission after lobectomy for lung cancer. Ann Surg 2019;1. Available at: http://insights.ovid.com/crossref?an=00000658-900000000-94927. Accessed November 16, 2019.

19. Jiang L, Jiang G, Zhu Y, et al. Risk factors predisposing to prolonged air leak after video-assisted thoracoscopic surgery for spontaneous pneumothorax. Ann Thorac Surg 2014.

20. Brunelli A, Monteverde M, Borri A, et al. Predictors of prolonged air leak after pulmonary lobectomy. Ann Thorac Surg 2004.

21. Ciccone AM, Meyers BF, Guthrie TJ, et al. Long-term outcome of bilateral lung volume reduction in 250 consecutive patients with emphysema. J Thorac Cardiovasc Surg 2003.

22. Zanotti G, Mitchell JD. Bronchopleural fistula and empyema after anatomic lung resection. Thorac Surg Clin 2015;25(4):421–7.

23. Olcmen A, Gunluoglu MZ, Demir A, et al. Role and outcome of surgery for pulmonary tuberculosis. Asian Cardiovasc Thorac Ann 2006.

24. Lang-Lazdunski L, Offredo C, Le Pimpec-Barthes F, et al. Pulmonary resection for Mycobacterium xenopi pulmonary infection. Ann Thorac Surg 2001.

25. Gómez-Caro A, Calvo MJR, Lanzas JT, et al. The approach of fused fissures with fissureless technique decreases the incidence of persistent air leak after lobectomy. Eur J Cardiothoracic Surg 2007.

26. Okereke I, Murthy SC, Alster JM, et al. Characterization and importance of air leak after lobectomy. Ann Thorac Surg 2005.

27. Lee L, Hanley SC, Robineau C, et al. Estimating the risk of prolonged air leak after pulmonary resection using a simple scoring system. J Am Coll Surg 2011.

28. Rivera C, Bernard A, Falcoz PE, et al. Characterization and prediction of prolonged air leak after pulmonary resection: A nationwide study setting up the index of prolonged air leak. Ann Thorac Surg 2011.

29. Algar FJ, Alvarez A, Aranda JL, et al. Prediction of early bronchopleural fistula after pneumonectomy: A multivariate analysis. Ann Thorac Surg 2001.

30. Wright CD, Wain JC, Mathisen DJ, et al. Postpneumonectomy bronchopleural fistula after sutured bronchial closure: Incidence, risk factors, and management. J Thorac Cardiovasc Surg 1996.

31. Viti A, Socci L, Congregado M, et al. The everlasting issue of prolonged air leaks after lobectomy for non-small cell lung cancer: A data-driven prevention planning model in the era of minimally invasive approaches. J Surg Oncol 2018.

32. Brunelli A, Varela G, Refai M, et al. A scoring system to predict the risk of prolonged air leak after lobectomy. Ann Thorac Surg 2010.

33. Pompili C, Falcoz PE, Salati M, et al. A risk score to predict the incidence of prolonged air leak after video-assisted thoracoscopic lobectomy: An analysis from the European Society of Thoracic Surgeons database. J Thorac Cardiovasc Surg 2017.

34. Orsini B, Baste JM, Gossot D, et al. Index of prolonged air leak score validation in case of video-assisted thoracoscopic surgery anatomical lung resection: Results of a nationwide study based on the French national thoracic database, EPITHOR. Eur J Cardiothoracic Surg 2015.

35. Attaar A, Winger DG, Luketich JD, et al. A clinical prediction model for prolonged air leak after pulmonary resection. J Thorac Cardiovasc Surg 2017.

36. Oh SG, Jung Y, Jheon S, et al. Postoperative air leak grading is useful to predict prolonged air leak after pulmonary lobectomy. J Cardiothorac Surg 2017.

37. Takamochi K, Imashimizu K, Fukui M, et al. Utility of objective chest tube management after pulmonary resection using a digital drainage system. Ann Thorac Surg 2017.

38. Brunelli A, Cassivi SD, Salati M, et al. Digital measurements of air leak flow and intrapleural pressures in the immediate postoperative period predict risk of prolonged air leak after pulmonary lobectomy. Eur J Cardio-thoracic Surg 2011.

39. Goto M, Aokage K, Sekihara K, et al. Prediction of prolonged air leak after lung resection using continuous log data of flow by digital drainage system. Gen Thorac Cardiovasc Surg 2019.

40. Yeung C, Ghazel M, French D, et al. Forecasting pulmonary air leak duration following lung surgery using transpleural airflow data from a digital pleural drainage device. J Thorac Dis 2018.

41. Rocco G, Brunelli A, Rocco R. Suction or nonsuction: how to manage a chest tube after pulmonary resection. Thorac Surg Clin 2017.

42. Cerfolio RJ, Bryant AS. The management of chest tubes after pulmonary resection. Thorac Surg Clin 2010.

43. Marshall MB, Deeb ME, Bleier JIS, et al. Suction vs water seal after pulmonary resection: A randomized prospective study. Chest 2002.

44. Cerfolio RJ, Bryant AS, Singh S, et al. The management of chest tubes in patients with a pneumothorax and an air leak after pulmonary resection. Chest 2005.

45. Coughlin SM, Emmerton-Coughlin HMA, Malthaner R. Management of chest tubes after pulmonary resection: A systematic review and meta-analysis. Can J Surg 2012.

46. Toloza EM, Harpole DH. Intraoperative techniques to prevent air leaks. Chest Surg Clin N Am 2002.

47. Varela G, Jiménez MF, Novoa N. Portable chest drainage systems and outpatient chest tube management. Thorac Surg Clin 2010.

48. Brims FJH, Maskell NA. Ambulatory treatment in the management of pneumothorax: A systematic review of the literature. Thorax 2013.

49. Towe CW, Khil A, Ho VP, et al. Early discharge after lung resection is safe: 10-year experience. J Thorac Dis 2018.

50. Linden PA, Perry Y, Worrell S, et al. Postoperative day 1 discharge after anatomic lung resection: A Society of Thoracic Surgeons database analysis. J Thorac Cardiovasc Surg 2019.

51. Rosen JE, Salazar MC, Dharmarajan K, et al. Length of stay from the hospital perspective: practice of early discharge is not associated with increased readmission risk after lung cancer surgery. Ann Surg 2017.

52. Reinersman JM, Allen MS, Blackmon SH, et al. Analysis of patients discharged from the hospital with a chest tube in place. Ann Thorac Surg 2018.

53. Jabłoński S, Kordiak J, Wcisło S, et al. Outcome of pleurodesis using different agents in management prolonged air leakage following lung resection. Clin Respir J 2018.

54. Özpolat B. Autologous blood patch pleurodesis in the management of prolonged air leak. Thorac Cardiovasc Surg 2010.

55. Travaline JM, McKenna RJ, De Giacomo T, et al. Treatment of persistent pulmonary air leaks using endobronchial valves. Chest 2009.

56. Gillespie CT, Sterman DH, Cerfolio RJ, et al. Endobronchial valve treatment for prolonged air leaks of the lung: A case series. Ann Thorac Surg 2011.

57. Reed MF, Gilbert CR, Taylor MD, et al. Endobronchial valves for challenging air leaks. Ann Thorac Surg 2015.

58. Firlinger I, Stubenberger E, Müller MR, et al. Endoscopic one-way valve implantation in patients with prolonged air leak and the use of digital air leak monitoring. Ann Thorac Surg 2013.

59. Cerfolio RJ. The incidence, etiology, and prevention of postresectional bronchopleural fistula. Semin Thorac Cardiovasc Surg 2001;13(1):3–7.

60. Nagahiro I, Aoe M, Sano Y, et al. Bronchopleural fistula after lobectomy for lung cancer. Asian Cardiovasc Thorac Ann 2007.

61. Sirbu H, Busch T, Aleksic I, et al. Bronchopleural fistula in the surgery of non-small cell lung cancer: incidence, risk factors, and management. Ann Thorac Cardiovasc Surg 2001;7(6):330–6.

62. Fuso L, Varone F, Nachira D, et al. Incidence and management of post-lobectomy and pneumonectomy bronchopleural fistula. Lung 2016.

63. Stern JB, Fournel L, Wyplosz B, et al. Early and delayed post-pneumonectomy empyemas: Microbiology, management and prognosis. Clin Respir J 2018.

64. Boudaya MS, Smadhi H, Zribi H, et al. Conservative management of postoperative bronchopleural fistulas. J Thorac Cardiovasc Surg 2013.

65. Zaheer S, Allen MS, Cassivi SD, et al. Postpneumonectomy empyema: results after the Clagett procedure. Ann Thorac Surg 2006.

66. Schneiter D, Grodzki T, Lardinois D, et al. Accelerated treatment of postpneumonectomy empyema: A binational long-term study. J Thorac Cardiovasc Surg 2008.

67. Alexiou C, Beggs D, Rogers ML, et al. Pneumonectomy for non-small cell lung cancer: Predictors of operative mortality and survival. Eur J Cardiothoracic Surg 2001.

68. Hu XF, Duan L, Jiang GN, et al. A clinical risk model for the evaluation of bronchopleural fistula in non-small cell lung cancer after pneumonectomy. Ann Thorac Surg 2013.

69. Jichen QV, Chen G, Jiang G, et al. Risk factor comparison and clinical analysis of early and late bronchopleural fistula after non-small cell lung cancer surgery. Ann Thorac Surg 2009.

70. Bribriesco A, Patterson GA. Management of postpneumonectomy bronchopleural fistula: from thoracoplasty to transsternal closure. Thorac Surg Clin 2018.

71. Brown LM, Vallieres E. 57 - Postsurgical empyema. In: LoCicero J, Feins RH, Colson YL, et al, editors. Shields' general thoracic surgery. 8th edition. Philadelphia: Lippincott Williams & Wilkins; 2019. p. 746–54.

72. Vallières E. Management of empyema after lung resections (pneumonectomy/lobectomy). Chest Surg Clin N Am 2002.

73. Wain JC. Management of late postpneumonectomy empyema and bronchopleural fistula. Chest Surg Clin N Am 1996;6(3):529–41. Available at: https://www.ncbi.nlm.nih.gov/pubmed/8818420. Accessed November 17, 2019.

74. Di Maio M, Perrone F, Deschamps C, et al. A meta-analysis of the impact of bronchial stump coverage

on the risk of bronchopleural fistula after pneumonectomy. Eur J Cardiothoracic Surg 2015;48(2): 196–200.

75. Pforr A, Pagès PB, Baste JM, et al. A predictive score for bronchopleural fistula established using the French database epithor. Ann Thorac Surg 2016.

76. Duque JL, Ramos G, Castrodeza J, et al. Early complications in surgical treatment of lung cancer: A prospective, multicenter study. Ann Thorac Surg 1997.

77. Li SJ, Fan J, Zhou J, et al. Diabetes mellitus and risk of bronchopleural fistula after pulmonary resections: a meta-analysis. Ann Thorac Surg 2016; 102(1):328–39.

78. Mazzella A, Pardolesi A, Maisonneuve P, et al. Bronchopleural fistula after pneumonectomy: risk factors and management, focusing on open-window thoracostomy. Semin Thorac Cardiovasc Surg 2018.

79. Puri V, Tran A, Bell JM, et al. Completion pneumonectomy: outcomes for benign and malignant indications. Ann Thorac Surg 2013.

80. Okuda M, Go T, Yokomise H. Risk factor of bronchopleural fistula after general thoracic surgery: review article. Gen Thorac Cardiovasc Surg 2017.

81. Fujimoto T, Zaboura G, Fechner S, et al. Completion pneumonectomy: current indications, complications, and results. J Thorac Cardiovasc Surg 2001.

82. Al-Kattan K, Goldstraw P. Completion pneumonectomy: indications and outcome. J Thorac Cardiovasc Surg 1995.

83. Miller DL, Deschamps C, Jenkins GD, et al. Completion pneumonectomy: Factors affecting operative mortality and cardiopulmonary morbidity. Ann Thorac Surg 2002.

84. Hamaji M, Chen-Yoshikawa TF, Date H. Completion pneumonectomy and auto-transplantation for bronchopleural fistula. J Thorac Cardiovasc Surg 2019.

85. Shapiro M, Swanson SJ, Wright CD, et al. Predictors of major morbidity and mortality after pneumonectomy utilizing the society for thoracic surgeons general thoracic surgery database. Ann Thorac Surg 2010.

86. Rivera C, Arame A, Pricopi C, et al. Pneumonectomy for benign disease: Indications and postoperative outcomes, a nationwide study. Eur J Cardiothoracic Surg 2015.

87. Reed CE. Pneumonectomy for chronic infection: Fraught with danger? Ann Thorac Surg 1995.

88. Kobayashi S, Karube Y, Nishihira M, et al. Postoperative pyothorax a risk factor for acute exacerbation of idiopathic interstitial pneumonia following lung cancer resection. Gen Thorac Cardiovasc Surg 2016.

89. Siegenthaler MP, Pisters KM, Merriman KW, et al. Preoperative chemotherapy for lung cancer does not increase surgical morbidity. Ann Thorac Surg 2001.

90. Li S, Fan J, Liu J, et al. Neoadjuvant therapy and risk of bronchopleural fistula after lung cancer surgery: A systematic meta-analysis of 14 912 patients. Jpn J Clin Oncol 2016.

91. Yamamoto R, Tada H, Kishi A, et al. Effects of preoperative chemotherapy and radiation therapy on human bronchial blood flow. J Thorac Cardiovasc Surg 2000.

92. Inui K, Takahashi Y, Hasegawa S, et al. Effect of preoperative irradiation on wound healing after bronchial anastomosis in mongrel dogs. J Thorac Cardiovasc Surg 1993.

93. Hollaus PH, Lax F, Janakiev D, et al. Endoscopic treatment of postoperative bronchopleural fistula: Experience with 45 cases. Ann Thorac Surg 1998.

94. Tsunezuka Y, Sato H, Tsukioka T, et al. A new instrument for endoscopic gluing for bronchopleural fistulae. Ann Thorac Surg 1999.

95. Stratakos G, Zuccatosta L, Porfyridis I, et al. Silver nitrate through flexible bronchoscope in the treatment of bronchopleural fistulae. J Thorac Cardiovasc Surg 2009.

96. Yamamoto S, Endo S, Minegishi K, et al. Polyglycolic acid mesh occlusion for postoperative bronchopleural fistula. Asian Cardiovasc Thorac Ann 2015.

97. Han X, Yin M, Li L, et al. Customized airway stenting for bronchopleural fistula after pulmonary resection by interventional technique: single-center study of 148 consecutive patients. Surg Endosc 2018.

98. Litle VR. Management of post-pneumonectomy bronchopleural fistula: a roadmap for rescue. Semin Thorac Cardiovasc Surg 2018.

99. Gómez JMN, Carbajo MC, Concha DV, et al. Conservative treatment of post-lobectomy bronchopleural fistula. Interact Cardiovasc Thorac Surg 2012.

100. Park JS, Eom JS, Choi SH, et al. Use of a serratus anterior musculocutaneous flap for surgical obliteration of a bronchopleural fistula. Interact Cardiovasc Thorac Surg 2015.

101. Massera F, Robustellini M, Della Pona C, et al. Open window thoracostomy for pleural empyema complicating partial lung resection. Ann Thorac Surg 2009;87. https://doi.org/10.1016/j.athoracsur.2008.12.003.

102. Regnard JF, Alifano M, Puyo P, et al. Open window thoracostomy followed by intrathoracic flap transposition in the treatment of empyema complicating pulmonary resection. J Thorac Cardiovasc Surg 2000.

103. Clagett OT, Geraci JE. A procedure for the management of postpneumonectomy empyema. J Thorac Cardiovasc Surg 1963.

104. Babu AN, Mitchell JD. Technique of muscle flap harvest for intrathoracic use. Oper Tech Thorac Cardiovasc Surg 2010.

105. Anderson TM, Miller JI. Use of pleura, azygos vein, pericardium, and muscle flaps in tracheobronchial surgery. Ann Thorac Surg 1995.

106. Taghavi S, Marta GM, Lang G, et al. Bronchial stump coverage with a pedicled pericardial flap: An effective method for prevention of postpneumonectomy bronchopleural fistula. Ann Thorac Surg 2005.

107. Anderson TM, Miller JI. Surgical technique and application of pericardial fat pad and pericardiophrenic grafts. Ann Thorac Surg 1995.

108. Fricke A, Bannasch H, Klein HF, et al. Pedicled and free flaps for intrathoracic fistula management. Eur J Cardiothorac Surg 2017.

109. Shrager JB, Wain JC, Wright CD, et al. Omentum is highly effective in the management of complex cardiothoracic surgical problems. J Thorac Cardiovasc Surg 2003.

110. Boulton BJ, Force S. The technique of omentum harvest for intrathoracic use. Oper Tech Thorac Cardiovasc Surg 2010.

111. D'Andrilli A, Ibrahim M, Andreetti C, et al. Transdiaphragmatic Harvesting of the Omentum Through Thoracotomy for Bronchial Stump Reinforcement. Ann Thorac Surg 2009.

112. Begum SSS, Papagiannopoulos K. The use of vacuum-assisted wound closure therapy in thoracic operations. Ann Thorac Surg 2012.

113. Karapinar K, Saydam Ö, Metin M, et al. Experience with vacuum-assisted closure in the management of postpneumonectomy empyema: an analysis of eight cases. Thorac Cardiovasc Surg 2016.

114. Ginsberg RJ, Saborio DV. Management of the recalcitrant postpneumonectomy bronchopleural fistula: The transsternal transpericardial approach. Semin Thorac Cardiovasc Surg 2001.

115. Galetta D, Spaggiari L. Video-thoracoscopic management of postpneumonectomy empyema. Thorac Cardiovasc Surg 2018.

116. Scarci M, Abah U, Solli P, et al. EACTS expert consensus statement for surgical management of pleural empyema. Eur J Cardiothoracic Surg 2015.

117. Leiter N, Pickering EM, Sangwan YS, et al. Intrapleural therapy for empyema in the setting of a bronchopleural fistula: a novel use of an intrabronchial valve. Ann Thorac Surg 2018.

118. Ding M, Gao YD, Zeng XT, et al. Endobronchial one-way valves for treatment of persistent air leaks: a systematic review. Respir Res 2017.

119. Kalatoudis H, Nikhil M, Zeid F, et al. Bronchopleural fistula resolution with endobronchial valve placement and liberation from mechanical ventilation in acute respiratory distress syndrome: a case series. Case Rep Crit Care 2017.

120. Brichon PY, Poquet C, Arvieux C, et al. Successful treatment of a life-threatening air leakage, complicating severe abdominal sepsis, with a one-way endobronchial valve. Interact Cardiovasc Thorac Surg 2012.

121. Fischer W, Feller-Kopman D, Shah A, et al. Endobronchial valve therapy for pneumothorax as a bridge to lung transplantation. J Hear Lung Transplant 2012.

Management of Complications After Esophagectomy

Jonathan C. Yeung, MD, PhD, FRCSC

KEYWORDS

- Esophagectomy • Complications • Esophageal cancer

KEY POINTS

- Esophagectomy is a complex operation with many potential complications.
- Early recognition of complication is vital to patient survival.
- Minimally invasive approaches for managing complications are emerging.

INTRODUCTION

Surgical resection remains a mainstay in curative-intent treatment of esophageal cancer. Esophagectomy is a complex operation, however, with myriad potential complications. Moreover, esophagectomy itself is a heterogenous group of operations with different approaches and anastomoses, each with its own side-effect profile. In a recent analysis of the multinational and standardized online database by the Esophageal Complications Consensus Group (ECCG), the incidence of complications was 59% with severe complications, as defined by a Clavien-Dindo grade greater than IIIB occurring in 17.2%.[1,2] Clearly, esophagectomy remains fraught with complication, and management thereof is vital. Improved management of these postoperative complications, however, has led to improved survival rates over the past 30 years.[3] This article reviews common surgical complications and their management.

ANASTOMOTIC LEAK

The most pressing concern after esophagectomy is leak at the gastroesophageal anastomosis. Early identification of leaks provides the best opportunity to minimize morbidity and mortality from a historically mortal complication.[4]

Risk Factors

Usually, leaks arise as a result of ischemia at the anastomosis, preventing adequate healing. The gastroesophageal anastomosis is particularly susceptible because the gastric conduit relies on the right gastroepiploic vessel as the sole source of blood supply, and careful preservation of this vessel during creation of the gastric conduit is paramount. This vessel, however, does not reach high onto the fundus where the anastomosis is created, and thus anastomosis viability requires adequate submucosal microvasculature from the right gastroepiploic vessel to the tip of the conduit.[5] Consequently, where the anastomosis is situated affects the leak rate. Anastomoses in the neck generally are associated with a higher risk of leak owing to the longer gastric conduit required and the higher amount of tension. Randomized controlled trials by Chasseray and colleagues,[6] Walther and colleagues,[7] and Okuyama and colleagues[8] all trended toward higher leak rates in the neck. In a review of the Society of Thoracic Surgeons database, Kassis and colleagues[9] showed a cervical anastomotic leak rate of 12.3% versus 9.3% in the chest, which is comparable to the ECCG leak rate of 11.4% for all-comers.

Toronto General Hospital, 200 Elizabeth Street 9N-983, Toronto, Ontario M5G 2C4, Canada
E-mail address: jonathan.yeung@uhn.ca

Thorac Surg Clin 30 (2020) 359–366
https://doi.org/10.1016/j.thorsurg.2020.04.002
1547-4127/20/© 2020 Elsevier Inc. All rights reserved.

Apart from where the anastomosis is located, how the anastomosis is formed also is diverse. Some surgeons prefer a hand-sewn anastomosis, others a stapled anastomosis either by circular stapler or by linear stapler. Blackmon and colleagues[10] retrospectively compared these 3 techniques and concluded that stapler techniques result in lower rates of stricture, but no difference in leak rates were identified. Wang and colleagues[11] subsequently performed a randomized controlled trial in 155 patients and demonstrated no difference in leak rates but a lower level of stricture using a linear stapler. Meta-analyses exploring this issue similar do not show any difference in leak rates between these methods, with the exception of perhaps more stricturing with circular stapler.[12,13] Overall, there is no apparent best technique for anastomosis construction.

In general, surgeons create a gastric conduit tube along the greater curve rather than utilize the whole stomach as a conduit. This is thought to help drainage of the conduit as well as to prevent thoracic stomach syndrome, where a distended stomach in the chest results in physiology similar to that of tension pneumothorax. The ideal width of this conduit, however, remains debated. Barbera and colleagues[14] showed that the narrower the conduit, the faster the emptying. Tubes that are narrower than 4 cm, however, are thought to affect the submucosal vessels and lead to conduit tip ischemia; however, this has not been demonstrated in randomized controlled trials. Tabira and colleagues[15] compared a subtotal stomach to a narrow gastric conduit, with 22 patients in each group, and Zhang and colleagues[16] compared a whole stomach conduit to a narrow gastric tube, with 52 patient in each group, and neither study showed a difference in leak rates but neither narrow tube was less than 4 cm. Other retrospective studies are conflicting in their conclusions.[17–19] Overall, conduit width down to approximately 4 cm does not seem to affect leak rate. Narrower or focally narrower conduits less than 4 cm may disturb the submucosal vessels and cause conduit tip ischemia but no formal study has shown this because likely no surgeon routinely uses conduits narrower than 4 cm.

Given that the stomach is devascularized and left to survive on the right gastroepiploic vessel at the time of conduit construction and anastomosis, a strategy to divide the vessels prior to conduit construction and anastomosis was devised as a form of ischemic preconditioning of the stomach. Two approaches have been described, one using arterial embolization and another using laparoscopic division of the vessels.[20,21] Arterial embolization showed less reduction in blood flow at the anastomotic site and lower leak rates but was complicated by splenic infarction and pancreatitis. Laparoscopic division allowed simultaneously for additional staging and lymph node dissection but meant that esophagectomy would need to occur in an operated field. Depending on the interval between laparoscopic intervention and esophagectomy, leak rates were lower or even higher, with 2 weeks the apparent minimum for benefit. A meta-analysis subsequently has been performed, demonstrating some minor reduction in leak rate from 14.1% to 8.8% but did not reach statistical significance.[22] Overall, there appears to be no strong benefit in small series and, given the logistical complexity and additional procedural risk, it does not appear that this approach is warranted.

Intraoperative vascular assessment is another strategy for assessment of the conduit. Use of intravenous indocyanine green dye and a near-infrared camera allows for real-time visualization of gastric conduit perfusion.[23] Small retrospective studies show this to be promising method to better situate the anastomosis.[24–26] A recent meta-analysis of the available literature supports the technique as being safe and as aiding in reducing leak; however, the quality of many of the articles was limited by small numbers and absence of a nonexposed cohort.[27] For now, it appears that use of intraoperative assessment may be helpful but further large-scale studies will be required to examine if anastomotic leak rates truly can be impacted.

Diagnosis

Early recognition of anastomotic leak is critical. In some cases, the leak will be apparent, that is, saliva or bile out a drain. In many cases, however, clinical presentation is subtle and any deviation from usual postoperative course should be cause for consideration of an anastomotic leak. Leaks can present as tachycardia, new atrial fibrillation, pain, respiratory compromise, and delirium, among others. It is important to never simply attribute something, such as atrial fibrillation or delirium, as a matter of postoperative course without consideration that a leak is the underlying cause. Anastomotic failures can be investigated in a variety of ways, each with its own pros and cons.[28] CT scan with oral contrast allows for identification of a leak by extraluminal contrast or air and also allows for assessment of collections and potential for drainage. Gastrograffin with or without barium swallow is most sensitive but does not allow for much assessment of surrounding structures. Endoscopic assessment allows for direct visualization of the defect and evaluation of the viability of the conduit and potentially allows for therapeutic intervention.

Management

Once a leak is identified, the extent of the leak needs to be assessed. Minor contained leaks, where a patient is clinically stable, can simply be observed for deterioration or treated with antibiotics, nasogastric decompression of the conduit, and distal enteral or parenteral nutrition. More significant leaks in the neck can be managed by opening the neck incision and placing drains to obtain source control. These drains can be shortened over the next few weeks as the defect heals. Major leaks in the chest are more challenging to deal with but follow the principles of source control. Collections need to be drained, the lung decorticated, and ongoing soilage of the chest controlled. In some cases, percutaneous drains are adequate to obtain source control. In more significant leaks, operative assessment may be required to assess whether the leak is from the anastomosis itself or along the gastric staple line. If the conduit is largely healthy, the defect can be reclosed and buttressed with vascularized tissue. The advent of minimally invasive approaches means that many muscle flaps remain available to the surgeon in the event of a leak, such as intercostal, serratus, or latissimus, and care during thoracotomy to protect potential flaps are needed.

Endoscopic stenting instead of operative repair of the leak more recently has been added to the management armamentarium. In this strategy, self-expanding fully covered metal stents are placed across the anastomotic defect to prevent further soilage of the thoracic cavity. It is important to remember that stenting is meant only to replace the operative closure of the leak. Drainage of existing collections for source control remains important. One major issue is that stents largely are designed to expand against strictures. In an esophagogastric anastomosis, the esophagus is of normal caliber but the conduit usually is larger. Thus, although the proximal flared portion of the stent may stay within the esophagus, the distal flared portion may not be large enough for the conduit, leading to inadequate sealing of the leak due to reflux of conduit contents behind the stent. Additional stents may be required to obtain a watertight seal for adequate source control. Another issue that can occur is the high propensity for stent migration because only the proximal flared portion can hold the fully covered stent in place. Thus, the largest fully covered double flared

stent should be chosen to avoid this issue, and clips on the esophageal side may be required. Multiple series have been published demonstrating the success of such a strategy.[29,30] A large series by Plum and colleagues[31] of 70 patients over 10 years demonstrated a sealing success rate of 70%, with a median treatment time of 28 days. Complications occurred in approximately 30% of cases in the forms of stenosis, stent migration, persistence of leakage, and perforation/esophago-airway fistula. Survival was 87% in patients who received a stent. Factors predictive of success were not identified in this study; thus, whom to stent remains subject to clinical judgment.

Recently, an alternative to self-expanding metal stents in the form of endoscopic vacuum therapy has been developed for the treatment of leaks. Continuous negative pressure is applied to the defect and cavity via a sponge placed endoscopically and attached to a nasogastric tube. de Moura and colleagues[32] describe a few methods of creating such a device. This is changed every 3 days to 4 days until the cavity is closed by granulation. This avoids some of the difficulties with stenting, such as incomplete occlusion of the leak and stent migration, and has the additional benefit of actively promoting wound healing by drainage of infected fluid and induction of granulation tissue. It can be resource-intensive, however, requiring scheduled dressing changes in an endoscopic suite or operating room setting. In small cohorts, success in closing anastomotic leaks have been approximately 80% to 90%, with a stricture rate of approximately 5% to 10%.[33–35] Also, in small cohorts, vacuum therapy has been shown superior to stents.[36–38] Endoscopic vacuum therapy is a potential strategy to accelerate healing of leaks.

CONDUIT NECROSIS

The most devastating leak is that caused by conduit necrosis, where the blood supply to the conduit is inadvertently interrupted and the conduit no longer is viable. This usually is recognized by a critically ill patient in septic shock but occasionally can present with unexplained fever, tachycardia, and delirium similar to that of a leak. As with an anastomotic leak, high clinical suspicion is needed and mortality can reach 90% with this condition.[39] After urgent resuscitation and antibiotics, evaluation should proceed in the operating room. Diagnosis of the necrotic conduit should begin with endoscopy in the operating room. Resection of the conduit then should occur with formation of an end esophagostomy. The longest possible length of residual esophagus should be preserved at this time to assist with future reconstruction and to better palliate the esophagostomy; an end esophagostomy situated on the chest can be hidden under clothes, and stoma appliances are secured more easily. A feeding enterotomy should be considered if not present and if the clinical status permits. After resolution of sepsis and optimization of nutrition, reconstruction can be performed. Conduit options after a necrotic gastric conduit include colon interposition and supercharged jejunal interposition in the substernal position.[40,41] In both cases, resection of the left hemimanubrium, clavicle, and first rib is needed to prevent obstruction and, when supercharging is required, to perform the vascular anastomoses.

CONDUIT-AIRWAY FISTULA

Another devastating complication that can occur in the setting of an anastomotic leak is a fistula between the anastomosis and the airway.[42] In the neck, the trachea is involved, and, in the chest, the trachea, carina, or either main bronchus could be involved. Airway injury during over-dissection may predispose a patient to such a fistula, but an undrained leak causing inflammation and digestion by gastric juices still may create an airway fistula. Stents used to treat leaks have eroded into the airway but may be a result of inadequate drainage rather than the expansile force of the stent.

Endoscopic approaches to repair these fistulae include the use of fibrin glue and Vicryl plugs, but, in 2 patients with airway-conduit fistulae, only 1 healed with this approach.[43] Clips to reapproximate such fistulae also have been attempted but, apart from a case report of a conduit to bronchial fistula, no large series of success have been reported.[44,45]

Another endoscopic strategy is the use of stents, esophageal, airway, or both to cover the defect. In a series of 6 patients by Schweigert and colleagues[46] with conduit-airway fistula, 2 underwent esophageal stenting, 1 underwent airway stenting, and 1 had both esophageal and airway stenting. Three of the 4 cases achieved definitive closure of the fistula after 6 weeks. The remainder of the patients were unable to undergo stenting due to an ischemic conduit and instead had resection of the conduit, repair and coverage of the airway defect with vascularized tissue, and end esophagostomy. Unfortunately, all died as a result of septic shock.

Endoscopic treatments appear to defy the surgical principles of fistula repair, that is, division of fistula, repair of both defects, and interposition of vascularized tissue. Small series, however, have demonstrated success in selected cases without conduit necrosis, likely reflecting the acute nature of the inflammatory process and lack of fistula epithelialization. Decision making during this complication is challenging. Source control is paramount, because ongoing soilage of the lungs and mediastinum propagates sepsis and obviates any chance for survival. Surgical source control by repairing the fistula during septic shock, however, is risky. Balakrishnan and colleagues[47] reviewed a single-center series of surgical management of conduit-airway fistula in 11 patients. Of the 3 deaths, 2 were performed in the early postoperative period (<2 weeks). In cases of conduit necrosis, the decision is clear that the dead viscera must be resected. In cases of leak, however, if rapid source control can be achieved with a stent, this may allow the patient to resolve the sepsis before definitive treatment. Moreover, as evidenced by some small series, closure of the fistula can sometimes occur simply with stenting.[48]

CHYLOTHORAX

Owing to the course of the thoracic duct close to the esophagus, inadvertent thoracic duct injury occurs approximately 4% of the time according to the ECCG, leading to chylothorax.[1] Although chyle generally is milky in color, the lack of fat intake in the early postoperative period can result in a clear liquid. Thus, chyle leak should be considered when large volumes of fluid are being drained in the early postoperative period. A pleural fluid triglyceride level greater than 110 mg/dL is chemical confirmation of the chylothorax.

Conservative management generally is attempted first in postoperative chylothorax. Principles include drainage to re-expand the lung and to assess daily volume of leakage, nutritional support, and medication to reduce chyle flow. In the postoperative esophagectomy population, feeding in the postoperative period involves feeding jejunostomy or total parenteral nutrition. Jejunal feeds should be switched to a high-protein, low-fat formulation with medium-chain triglycerides.[48] Avoidance of long-chain triglycerides avoids their breakdown into monoglycerides and free fatty acids that are carried as chylomicrons in chyle. Octreotide can be attempted to decrease the flow of chyle by decreasing foregut secretions.

For esophagectomy, early reintervention for thoracic duct ligation should be considered because it is most likely that the thoracic duct itself was injured rather than any peripheral branch and unlikely to resolve. In addition, the increased use of induction radiation reduces the ability of the lymphatic network to heal. Lagarde and colleagues[49] used a cutoff of 2 L after 2 days to indicate surgery, and Reisenauer and colleagues[50] recommend surgery for an output of greater than 1.1 L over 24 hours at any point. Thus, if drainage does not fall below 1 L/24 hours within 1 day to 2 days of initiating conservative management, surgical intervention should be considered. The thoracic duct can carry up to 4 L of lymphocyte, lipid, and protein-rich chyle daily; thus, delay in sealing the chyle leak can result in malnutrition and immunodeficiency and affect healing of the anastomosis and delay postoperative recovery.

Surgical ligation of the duct requires rethoracotomy or thoracoscopy. To facilitate identification of the duct, a bolus of high-fat material, such as cream or oil, or through the jejunostomy tube no longer than 30 minutes to 60 minutes prior to operation can be helpful to make the chyle appear more opaque. Thoracic duct embolization is increasingly available as a nonsurgical option. Percutaneous embolization was successful in approximately of 80% of cases in small series.[51,52] Thoracic duct embolization was shown to be a useful technique after failed surgical thoracic duct ligation and identified aberrant duct anatomy, collaterals, or incomplete ligation causing failure.[53] In small series, lymphangiography alone also was shown to be successful.[54–56] With increasing experience, this may become the first line of treatment, but the complication profile remains to be fully defined. For now, in an otherwise fit patient, surgical treatment seems to be the best first option, but institutional expertise guides treatment.

Given the low risk of thoracic duct clipping, routine prophylactic duct ligation at the time of surgery may prevent the development of chylothorax. Guo and colleagues[57] performed a retrospective cohort study and showed that routine ligation of the duct reduced chylothorax rates from 10% to 1.5% in approximately 70 patients per group, and Dougenis and colleagues[58] reduced the rate from 9% to 2.1%. The approximately 10% rate is higher, however, than in other reported series. Lin and colleagues[59] compared routine ligation to selective ligation based on a bolus of olive oil given orally preoperatively and showed a reduction of chyle leak from 10% in the routinely ligated group to 0% in the selective group. The 10% leak rate in the routine ligation group seems high in contrast to the other studies. Reisenauer and colleagues[61] showed no difference (4% to 4%) but only a small number of patients underwent prophylactic ligation.

RECURRENT LARYNGEAL NERVE INJURY

The incidence of recurrent laryngeal nerve injury is 3.5%, according to the ECCG.[1] Due to its anatomic location, it is most at risk with a cervical anastomosis and with a 3-field lymph node dissection. Injury to the nerve can occur as a result of traction, overdissection, or transection. Although many injuries result in only transient dysfunction, the dysfunction is during the immediate postoperative period, when risk is highest. To prevent injury, Orringer and colleagues[60] recommend the "compulsive avoidance" of using metal instruments in the neck and suggest finger retraction and dissection of the esophagus as ideal. The symptoms of recurrent laryngeal nerve injury are due to lateral displacement of the affected vocal cord. Hoarseness is the primary symptom, but the voice also can be affected by ineffectively cleared secretions pooling in the pyriform sinus. This difficulty in clearing secretions also predisposes to aspiration of food and saliva, leading to pneumonia. Finally, the inability to close the glottis disrupts the Valsalva mechanism and makes straining difficult.

Upon discovery of a hoarse voice postoperatively, speech and language pathology should be involved to evaluate swallowing as soon as a patient is cleared for diet from the esophagectomy perspective. Maneuvers, such as supraglottic swallowing, may help minimize aspiration during swallowing.[62] Treatment of the dysfunction requires the assistance of otolaryngology. Due to the often transient nature of the nerve dysfunction, the first intervention usually is an injection augmentation of the affected cord to move it into the midline.[63] This injection is temporary but mitigates dysphonia and dysphagia in the short term to await return of function of the recurrent laryngeal nerve. After 6 months, if there is no recovery, medialization laryngoplasty can be performed for more permanent medialization of the cord.[64]

SUMMARY

Esophagectomy, in all its varieties, remains a complex operation with high potential for postoperative complications. Understanding the causes of complications allows for both prevention and salvage of the patient when it does occur.

DISCLOSURE

The author has nothing to disclose.

REFERENCES

1. Low DE, Kuppusamy MK, Alderson D, et al. Benchmarking Complications Associated with Esophagectomy. Ann Surg 2019;269(2):291–8.
2. Dindo D, Demartines N, Clavien PA. Classification of surgical complications: a new proposal with

evaluation in a cohort of 6336 patients and results of a survey. Ann Surg 2004;240(2):205–13.

3. Ruol A, Castoro C, Portale G, et al. Trends in management and prognosis for esophageal cancer surgery: twenty-five years of experience at a single institution. Arch Surg 2009;144(3):247–54 [discussion: 254].

4. Martin LW, Swisher SG, Hofstetter W, et al. Intrathoracic leaks following esophagectomy are no longer associated with increased mortality. Ann Surg 2005;242(3):392–9 [discussion: 399–402].

5. Liebermann-Meffert DM, Meier R, Siewert JR. Vascular anatomy of the gastric tube used for esophageal reconstruction. Ann Thorac Surg 1992;54(6):1110–5.

6. Chasseray VM, Kiroff GK, Buard JL, et al. Cervical or thoracic anastomosis for esophagectomy for carcinoma. Surg Gynecol Obstet 1989;169(1):55–62.

7. Walther B, Johansson J, Johnsson F, et al. Cervical or thoracic anastomosis after esophageal resection and gastric tube reconstruction: a prospective randomized trial comparing sutured neck anastomosis with stapled intrathoracic anastomosis. Ann Surg 2003;238(6):803–12 [discussion: 812–4].

8. Okuyama M, Motoyama S, Suzuki H, et al. Hand-sewn cervical anastomosis versus stapled intrathoracic anastomosis after esophagectomy for middle or lower thoracic esophageal cancer: a prospective randomized controlled study. Surg Today 2007;37(11):947–52.

9. Kassis ES, Kosinski AS, Ross P Jr, et al. Predictors of anastomotic leak after esophagectomy: an analysis of the society of thoracic surgeons general thoracic database. Ann Thorac Surg 2013;96(6):1919–26.

10. Blackmon SH, Correa AM, Wynn B, et al. Propensity-matched analysis of three techniques for intrathoracic esophagogastric anastomosis. Ann Thorac Surg 2007;83(5):1805–13 [discussion: 1813].

11. Wang WP, Gao Q, Wang KN, et al. A prospective randomized controlled trial of semi-mechanical versus hand-sewn or circular stapled esophagogastrostomy for prevention of anastomotic stricture. World J Surg 2013;37(5):1043–50.

12. Markar SR, Karthikesalingam A, Vyas S, et al. Hand-sewn versus stapled oesophago-gastric anastomosis: systematic review and meta-analysis. J Gastrointest Surg 2011;15(5):876–84.

13. Honda M, Kuriyama A, Noma H, et al. Hand-sewn versus mechanical esophagogastric anastomosis after esophagectomy: a systematic review and meta-analysis. Ann Surg 2013;257(2):238–48.

14. Barbera L, Solymosi N, Dubecz A, et al. [Effect of site and width of stomach tube after esophageal resection on gastric emptying]. Zentralbl Chir 1994;119(4):240–4.

15. Tabira Y, Sakaguchi T, Kuhara H, et al. The width of a gastric tube has no impact on outcome after esophagectomy. Am J Surg 2004;187(3):417–21.

16. Zhang C, Wu QC, Hou PY, et al. Impact of the method of reconstruction after oncologic oesophagectomy on quality of life–a prospective, randomised study. Eur J Cardiothorac Surg 2011;39(1):109–14.

17. Shu YS, Sun C, Shi WP, et al. Tubular stomach or whole stomach for esophagectomy through cervico-thoraco-abdominal approach: a comparative clinical study on anastomotic leakage. Ir J Med Sci 2013;182(3):477–80.

18. Shen Y, Wang H, Feng M, et al. The effect of narrowed gastric conduits on anastomotic leakage following minimally invasive oesophagectomy. Interact Cardiovasc Thorac Surg 2014;19(2):263–8.

19. Collard JM, Tinton N, Malaise J, et al. Esophageal replacement: gastric tube or whole stomach? Ann Thorac Surg 1995;60(2):261–6 [discussion: 267].

20. Akiyama S, Ito S, Sekiguchi H, et al. Preoperative embolization of gastric arteries for esophageal cancer. Surgery 1996;120(3):542–6.

21. Nguyen NT, Longoria M, Sabio A, et al. Preoperative laparoscopic ligation of the left gastric vessels in preparation for esophagectomy. Ann Thorac Surg 2006;81(6):2318–20.

22. Markar SR, Arya S, Karthikesalingam A, et al. Technical factors that affect anastomotic integrity following esophagectomy: systematic review and meta-analysis. Ann Surg Oncol 2013;20(13):4274–81.

23. Rino Y, Yukawa N, Sato T, et al. Visualization of blood supply route to the reconstructed stomach by indocyanine green fluorescence imaging during esophagectomy. BMC Med Imaging 2014;14:18.

24. Karampinis I, Ronellenfitsch U, Mertens C, et al. Indocyanine green tissue angiography affects anastomotic leakage after esophagectomy. A retrospective, case-control study. Int J Surg 2017;48:210–4.

25. Kitagawa H, Namikawa T, Iwabu J, et al. Assessment of the blood supply using the indocyanine green fluorescence method and postoperative endoscopic evaluation of anastomosis of the gastric tube during esophagectomy. Surg Endosc 2018;32(4):1749–54.

26. Ohi M, Toiyama Y, Mohri Y, et al. Prevalence of anastomotic leak and the impact of indocyanine green fluorescein imaging for evaluating blood flow in the gastric conduit following esophageal cancer surgery. Esophagus 2017;14(4):351–9.

27. Slooter MD, Eshuis WJ, Cuesta MA, et al. Fluorescent imaging using indocyanine green during esophagectomy to prevent surgical morbidity: a systematic review and meta-analysis. J Thorac Dis 2019;11(Suppl 5):S755–65.

28. Low DE. Diagnosis and management of anastomotic leaks after esophagectomy. J Gastrointest Surg 2011;15(8):1319–22.

29. Schweigert M, Solymosi N, Dubecz A, et al. Endoscopic stent insertion for anastomotic leakage following oesophagectomy. Ann R Coll Surg Engl 2013;95(1):43–7.

30. Schaheen L, Blackmon SH, Nason KS. Optimal approach to the management of intrathoracic esophageal leak following esophagectomy: a systematic review. Am J Surg 2014;208(4):536–43.

31. Plum PS, Herbold T, Berlth F, et al. Outcome of self-expanding metal stents in the treatment of anastomotic leaks after ivor lewis esophagectomy. World J Surg 2019;43(3):862–9.

32. de Moura DTH, de Moura B, Manfredi MA, et al. Role of endoscopic vacuum therapy in the management of gastrointestinal transmural defects. World J Gastrointest Endosc 2019;11(5):329–44.

33. Ahrens M, Schulte T, Egberts J, et al. Drainage of esophageal leakage using endoscopic vacuum therapy: a prospective pilot study. Endoscopy 2010;42(9):693–8.

34. Wedemeyer J, Schneider A, Manns MP, et al. Endoscopic vacuum-assisted closure of upper intestinal anastomotic leaks. Gastrointest Endosc 2008; 67(4):708–11.

35. Schorsch T, Muller C, Loske G. Endoscopic vacuum therapy of anastomotic leakage and iatrogenic perforation in the esophagus. Surg Endosc 2013; 27(6):2040–5.

36. Brangewitz M, Voigtlander T, Helfritz FA, et al. Endoscopic closure of esophageal intrathoracic leaks: stent versus endoscopic vacuum-assisted closure, a retrospective analysis. Endoscopy 2013;45(6): 433–8.

37. Mennigen R, Harting C, Lindner K, et al. Comparison of Endoscopic Vacuum Therapy Versus Stent for Anastomotic Leak After Esophagectomy. J Gastrointest Surg 2015;19(7):1229–35.

38. Schniewind B, Schafmayer C, Voehrs G, et al. Endoscopic endoluminal vacuum therapy is superior to other regimens in managing anastomotic leakage after esophagectomy: a comparative retrospective study. Surg Endosc 2013;27(10):3883–90.

39. Urschel JD. Esophagogastrostomy anastomotic leaks complicating esophagectomy: a review. Am J Surg 1995;169(6):634–40.

40. Cerfolio RJ, Allen MS, Deschamps C, et al. Esophageal replacement by colon interposition. Ann Thorac Surg 1995;59(6):1382–4.

41. Blackmon SH, Correa AM, Skoracki R, et al. Supercharged pedicled jejunal interposition for esophageal replacement: a 10-year experience. Ann Thorac Surg 2012;94(4):1104–11 [discussion: 1111–3].

42. Bartels HE, Stein HJ, Siewert JR. Tracheobronchial lesions following oesophagectomy: prevalence, predisposing factors and outcome. Br J Surg 1998; 85(3):403–6.

43. Truong S, Bohm G, Klinge U, et al. Results after endoscopic treatment of postoperative upper gastrointestinal fistulas and leaks using combined Vicryl plug and fibrin glue. Surg Endosc 2004; 18(7):1105–8.

44. Nardella JE, Van Raemdonck D, Piessevaux H, et al. Gastro-tracheal fistula–unusual and life threatening complication after esophagectomy for cancer: a case report. J Cardiothorac Surg 2009;4:69.

45. Kordzadeh A, Syllaios A, Davakis S, et al. Over-the-scope-clip treatment of gastrobronchial fistula following minimally invasive oesophagectomy: a novel approach. J Surg Case Rep 2019;2019(8): rjz229.

46. Schweigert M, Dubecz A, Beron M, et al. Management of anastomotic leakage-induced tracheobronchial fistula following oesophagectomy: the role of endoscopic stent insertion. Eur J Cardiothorac Surg 2012;41(5):e74–80.

47. Balakrishnan A, Tapias L, Wright CD, et al. Surgical management of post-esophagectomy tracheo-bronchial-esophageal fistula. Ann Thorac Surg 2018; 106(6):1640–6.

48. Lambertz R, Holscher AH, Bludau M, et al. Management of Tracheo- or Bronchoesophageal Fistula After Ivor-Lewis Esophagectomy. World J Surg 2016; 40(7):1680–7.

49. Jensen GL, Mascioli EA, Meyer LP, et al. Dietary modification of chyle composition in chylothorax. Gastroenterology 1989;97(3):761–5.

50. Lagarde SM, Omloo JM, de Jong K, et al. Incidence and management of chyle leakage after esophagectomy. Ann Thorac Surg 2005;80(2):449–54.

51. Reisenauer JS, Puig CA, Reisenauer CJ, et al. Treatment of Postsurgical Chylothorax. Ann Thorac Surg 2018;105(1):254–62.

52. Marthaller KJ, Johnson SP, Pride RM, et al. Percutaneous embolization of thoracic duct injury post-esophagectomy should be considered initial treatment for chylothorax before proceeding with open re-exploration. Am J Surg 2015;209(2):235–9.

53. Lambertz R, Chang DH, Hickethier T, et al. Ultrasound-guided lymphangiography and interventional embolization of chylous leaks following esophagectomy. Innov Surg Sci 2019;4(3):85–90.

54. Nadolski GJ, Itkin M. Lymphangiography and thoracic duct embolization following unsuccessful thoracic duct ligation: Imaging findings and outcomes. J Thorac Cardiovasc Surg 2018;156(2): 838–43.

55. Tamura T, Kubo N, Yamamoto A, et al. Cervical chylous leakage following esophagectomy that was successfully treated by intranodal lipiodol lymphangiography: a case report. BMC Surg 2017; 17(1):20.

56. Atie M, Dunn G, Falk GL. Chlyous leak after radical oesophagectomy: Thoracic duct lymphangiography

and embolisation (TDE)-A case report. Int J Surg Case Rep 2016;23:12–6.

57. Yamamoto M, Miyata H, Yamasaki M, et al. Chylothorax after esophagectomy cured by intranodal lymphangiography: a case report. Anticancer Res 2015;35(2):891–5.

58. Guo W, Zhao YP, Jiang YG, et al. Prevention of postoperative chylothorax with thoracic duct ligation during video-assisted thoracoscopic esophagectomy for cancer. Surg Endosc 2012;26(5):1332–6.

59. Dougenis D, Walker WS, Cameron EW, et al. Management of chylothorax complicating extensive esophageal resection. Surg Gynecol Obstet 1992; 174(6):501–6.

60. Orringer MB, Marshall B, Chang AC, et al. Two thousand transhiatal esophagectomies: changing trends, lessons learned. Ann Surg 2007;246(3): 363–72 [discussion: 372–4].

61. Lin Y, Li Z, Li G, et al. Selective en masse ligation of the thoracic duct to prevent chyle leak after esophagectomy. Ann Thorac Surg 2017;103(6):1802–7.

62. Aneas GC, Ricz HM, Mello-Filho FV, et al. Swallowing evaluation in patients with unilateral vocal fold immobility. Gastroenterol Res 2010;3(6):245–52.

63. Mallur PS, Rosen CA. Vocal fold injection: review of indications, techniques, and materials for augmentation. Clin Exp Otorhinolaryngol 2010;3(4): 177–82.

64. Daniero JJ, Garrett CG, Francis DO. Framework surgery for treatment of unilateral vocal fold paralysis. Curr Otorhinolaryngol Rep 2014;2(2):119–30.

Moving?

Make sure your subscription moves with you!

To notify us of your new address, find your **Clinics Account Number** (located on your mailing label above your name), and contact customer service at:

Email: journalscustomerservice-usa@elsevier.com

800-654-2452 (subscribers in the U.S. & Canada)
314-447-8871 (subscribers outside of the U.S. & Canada)

Fax number: 314-447-8029

Elsevier Health Sciences Division
Subscription Customer Service
3251 Riverport Lane
Maryland Heights, MO 63043

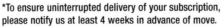
*To ensure uninterrupted delivery of your subscription, please notify us at least 4 weeks in advance of move.

ELSEVIER

Printed and bound by CPI Group (UK) Ltd, Croydon, CR0 4YY

08/05/2025

01864691-0012